DARE TO BE SEEN

From Stage Fright to Stage Presence

Ten Easy Steps to Turn your
Performance Anxiety into Authentic Power
with Transformational Hypnotherapy

Elisa Di Napoli

EDN Publishing
28 Carnegie Court EH8 9SN, Edinburgh, Scotland, UK

Disclaimer:

The advice and strategies found within may not be suitable for every situation. Results
cannot be guaranteed, and depend on personal response to hypnosis. We request that you
do not participate in hypnotherapy if you have any past or existing concerns about your
mental health. This work is sold with the understanding that neither the author nor the
publisher are held responsible for the results accrued from the advice in this book.

ISBN:978-1-9161797-1-4

This book is dedicated to my old friend and teacher, Angelo Marras.

You believed in me when I didn't. You really were an angel, just like your name suggests…

Acknowledgements

I want to extend a huge thank you to the following people:

My parents

My father, who has never been afraid to explore new horizons. His courage and determination have inspired me to do the same.

My mother, who has always encouraged me in my ideas, my music, and my skills. She is my biggest fan and her belief in me means the world to me.

My acquired family

My partner, Scott Murphy, who has been a pillar of strength and unwavering support like no other. He listened patiently, encouraged me, and made me endless cups of tea, occasionally reminding me to eat when I forgot to.

My ex-husband Chris Gilman, who read the manuscript and offered invaluable feedback. His vision and experience have been eye-opening and incredibly helpful.

My inspirations and teachers

Maureen Mulder, Ormond Mc Gill, Randal Churchill, Adam Eason and Mark Tyrrell, who are pioneers of hypnotherapy and have taught me to walk the talk and never stop learning. Also, Rachel Jayne Groover, who inspired me with her great teachings and coaching.

My clients

Too many to mention, who have taught me how to be a good therapist more than any book or course would. I especially would like to thank the kind people who have contributed to this book with their case studies. Your experience is helping others know it is possible to make change happen.

My readers and helpers

Em Strang, Mary Davidson, and Angelica Tsakmakidou for their comments and feedback. Their selfless support has meant more than I can say.

My music fans

Who have encouraged me to become a better performer, get out of my comfort zone, and keep going.

**DOWNLOAD the Dare to Be Seen
BONUS PACKAGE**

including a

**FREE AUDIOBOOK,
CHECKLIST, WORKBOOK and
ONLINE COURSE**

Templates, Training, Resources to Kickstart your Journey
into Authentic Confidence under the Spotlight!

TO DOWNLOAD GO TO
https://elisadinapoli.com/bonuses

CONTENTS

Foreword

Having had discussions with Elisa online previously, I first met her in person in my home town of Bournemouth when she was a student in my class. She was already very well experienced and qualified as a hypnotherapist and was seeking to continue developing. She relished doing so and continues to be a committed, tenacious, and reflective student of her subjects today.

The main tribute to her journey that I can offer up is that (as you'll read early on in this book) her story illustrates a battle with self-belief and confidence and yet she has become someone who knows herself and her own mind, and now readily shares her conviction for others to learn to do the same in this excellent book.

To the point whereby concepts I have taught whereby she sought a more in-depth understanding, or to disagree with, were confidently and willingly questioned by Elisa. Core concepts that I suggested she consider leaving behind, where she felt they had a depth of importance, she'd persist with and make them work for her, and some of them appear here in this book that I am writing the foreword to, which affords me a wry smile while writing. She never sought to simply confirm what she already knew, but would defend a process she believed offered value going forward.

You see, in addition to being an eclectic performance artist, Elisa has shared genuinely an equally diverse approach that she has found to be extremely effective, and I think you will too. However, you are likely to discover much more benefit on these pages if you also read between the lines of what is being written here.

Yes, you can apply the abundance of skills and adopt the strategies and processes, and you will derive a healthy degree of success. When you read deeper and detect the manner, the attitude, the striving for something more, then the content of this book will really sing to you and resonate with you profoundly.

Elisa's own journey with her confidence and self-belief is a fascinating one that culminates in a book rich with experience.

My experience has led me to a place whereby I'd never want to be too confident as a practitioner or as a lecturer or as a researcher as the slight self-doubt I still encounter on occasions keeps me sharp, keeps me striving to develop, keeps me humble and there is a tone of Elisa's humility and wisdom to her glowing self-belief that builds a foundation to this book that brings it all to life in ways you must not overlook.

There are ways Elisa prefers to do things, but the book is not telling you just to do them in rote fashion. The contents of the book are not like learning the correct pronunciation of her name. Instead, the attitude is one that can be modelled—not copied or mimicked but understood and then allowed to inspire you. She knows herself, and her message extends to one that encourages you to know yourself and then apply skills and adopt strategies, of which this book is filled to the brim with also.

Immerse and enjoy.

Yours with much love,
Adam Eason
Author, The Science of Self-Hypnosis: The Evidence-Based Way to Hypnotise Yourself
Principal, The Anglo European College of Therapeutic Hypnosis

INTRODUCTION

My Struggle with
Performance Anxiety
and How I've Overcome It

Although music is one of my biggest passions, I almost gave up my singing career at one point in my life because of performance anxiety. In this chapter, I want to tell you the story of how I managed, after many years of struggle, to overcome this issue once and for all.

My name is Elisa Di Napoli, but when I'm on stage, I call myself Elyssa Vulpes. The main reason is that when I first started my clinical practice, I felt embarrassed, scared, and sometimes even ashamed of also being a performer. The official reason was that I didn't want people to look me up on Facebook and find photos of me singing and playing drums and generally going wild at festivals. I was worried they'd lose trust in my abilities as a therapist, but I also felt too vulnerable to allow myself to be fully seen and heard, so I split my identity in two.

I'm telling you this, because every time we hide a part of ourselves for fear of rejection or embarrassment, we suffer and find less of that acceptance that we crave. Luckily, my commitment towards integrity, wholeness, and a sense of authenticity kept demanding I bring these two aspects of my life together—but for the longest time, I couldn't figure out how.

For many years before becoming a full-time therapist, I had tried to 'make it' as a musician but suffered from a bad case of the not-good-enough. I never felt comfortable with both self-promotion and public performances. This is because both have as their foundation a firm belief in our worthiness of being seen and heard. I never entirely gave up on my dreams, but when it became clear to me that I had "failed" at my goal of achieving fame and fortune, I decided to shift focus, and my passion for psychology and healing led to starting my own business.

Having a successful clinical practice helped me a lot in terms of developing a healthy dose of self-esteem, but after many years of dedicating myself to the business of serving others, I still felt a lack of balance in my life. I needed to rediscover my creativity so I could overcome my fears and limitations.

Fish don't know they are in the water, and in the same way, I could not see the obvious solution to my performance anxiety problem. Although I had been helping people with anxiety using hypnotherapy for years, it just never occurred to me that I could try it to overcome my performance anxiety. Instead, I went about it in all the wrong ways: I tried to drink wine before a gig, but it only made me feel sick and forget the chords of my songs. I tried Beta Blockers, but they made me feel strangely dissociated from my performance and my audience. Improv classes worked to keep me a little more 'in the moment', however I still felt like a wreck whenever I had to play my own songs.

I realised I needed to understand the mindset of those who were able to perform well despite their nerves. Would they feel nervous or distracted while playing? Would they always be thinking about the mistakes they could be making? Were they ever worried about what they imagined others were thinking of them? Or would they not be concerned at all with how they came across? Wouldn't it be more likely they just cared about the piece they were playing or the speech they were giving and were wholly immersed in its feeling and message? They seemed to be enjoying themselves, and that joy seemed to pass over onto the audience. I needed to feel the same way they did, and to do that, I needed to *think* the same way.

I knew that was something hypnotherapy could help with, so I sought the assistance of a colleague. A couple of sessions with him helped me realise that anxiety was at the core of my distracting thoughts, and that could be reduced by a mindset focussed on staying in the present. The sessions also addressed my concern with trying to focus on the enjoyment of the moment, rather than to fixate on perfectionism and judgment.

Although this approach helped, it didn't 'fix' me completely. I decided to get back to studying so I could approach the issue from every angle and find the best ways of resolving it. After doing a lot of research and helping many clients with this problem, I ended up developing an entire system that addressed all aspects of the question to make sure that even the most complex cases could be successfully treated.

At this point, I started thinking about writing a book and preparing an online course to teach others what I had discovered so that as many people as possible could benefit from it, but something kept stalling me. A question at the back of my mind demanded: who was I to write a book about performance anxiety?

I had not entirely overcome my fear, so I was just a fraud! I would be found out and publicly shamed! I hoped the problem would vanish in time, but of course, that didn't happen.

Finally, one day the obvious answer came to me: I had helped hundreds of people successfully deal with their issues in this area, and I already had all the tools I needed to leave my problems behind, but I just refused to use them, because I wanted *someone else* to save me.

The solution would be to actually *practice* the techniques outlined within my book. By taking responsibility, doing the work, and walking the talk, I could stop feeling like a fraud and transform into the performer I wanted to be. I would also be able to merge my two identities back together, revealing who I was and risking judgment, but becoming whole in the process.

I want this to become your success story, too. Because it is possible not only to be on stage and feel calm and confident, but also to look forward to it as an opportunity to be seen, heard, and to share your light with the world. So, let's jump right in and have some fun!

My Approach

Before I get into the details of this course, I want to make sure you understand why the techniques I use are effective. Here's how my approach is different and what makes it so successful.

Many books have been written on how to overcome performance anxiety. So, why should you trust my approach? My method is different because I will not just present you with theory, speculation, or even research on the matter. This book will not be simply an exposition of case studies and interviews, and won't just offer you some good advice. I also won't go into the details of the *content* of your 'performance' as that is beyond my area of expertise, and there are excellent books out there on the subject.

Instead, I am going to present you with a *practical* program that will guide you step by step to achieve the results you want. This approach is holistic, pragmatic, practical, progressive, and complete. Let me offer you my take on these terms.

Holistic

A "holistic" system considers the person as an integrated whole that is more than the sum of its parts. This method of treating the issue at hand takes into consideration how each part of a human being interacts with all the other parts.

I am alluding to your psychology, your feelings, your behaviour, your body, and your energy. This is because for you to change, you need to have the right mindset: you need to think the right thoughts and talk to yourself in the way a mindful and completely present performer does. You also need to feel like someone who enjoys being on stage.

Your energy needs to be in the right place, and finally you need to have the right experience of what it's like to give an excellent performance so you can do it again and again. In other words, your positive thoughts need to reinforce your positive feelings. This will change your energy, and as your energy changes, your body will be at its optimal level to allow positive experiences to be formed around performance. This, in turn, will reinforce the right mindset, which will feed the right feelings so you'll find yourself in a positively reinforcing spiral.

Pragmatic

I only use whatever has worked before with hundreds of clients. My approach is not dogmatic, and it combines the principles of Cognitive Behaviour Hypnotherapy, Human Givens Psychology, as well as Psychodynamic and Humanistic theories of psychology, which have been proven repeatedly to be effective in my clinical practice. What this means is that the body of work I am presenting looks at the issue of performance anxiety from different and complementary angles, leaving nothing out.

Cognitive behaviour theory is based on the idea that our thoughts determine our feelings and behaviour and that in turn, can influence our thinking. Negative thinking patterns and negative bias will create negative interpretations of reality, which give negative meanings to our experiences. These, in turn, produce negative feelings which create behaviours that reinforce the original negative thinking patterns.

For example, if you think that you are not good enough as a speaker, you will not feel confident on stage, which will lead you to give a poor performance. As a result, you are likely to judge your performance as below standard, which in turn will reinforce the original thought of you not being good enough.

This approach is complemented by **Human Givens Psychology[1],** which states that every behaviour serves the function of trying to meet the individual's emotional needs in a sometimes functional, sometimes

---

[1] For more info on this modality, I would suggest you visit https://www.hgi.org.uk/

dysfunctional way. When we understand what need the behaviour is trying to meet, we can answer it in a healthier way. The strategies I use involve promoting positive thinking as well as encouraging behaviours that serve a positive function in our life by helping us cope well in the present.

For example, you may have developed a drinking habit trying to cope with your nerves. The drinking behaviour serves the function of trying to help you relax. However, the need to stay calm is not being met in a functional way, since drinking may slow down your thinking, slur your words, and in the end, can cause you to develop a dependency. A more functional way of meeting this need would be to learn diaphragmatic breathing, which is proven to calm you down effectively.

Psychodynamic theory holds that past experiences shape how we behave in terms of both conscious and unconscious forces. Therefore, this book deals with the underlying causes of your fear of performing in public. When you allow emotions to be released, conflicts can be resolved, and events that caused the fear are reframed in a helpful light.

You may have suffered from traumatic experiences related to performance in the past. Perhaps you were shamed in public, or you may have felt extreme embarrassment while performing. This has caused you to subsequently fear similar situations. During a regressive hypnotherapy session, you would go back to the memories of these events to release unresolved emotions and reprocess them in a way that helps you move forward.

Humanistic theory believes that people seek to grow psychologically and are motivated by a wish to feel more fulfilled. They have free will and can choose their destiny consciously. It also holds that the way we interpret events is essential to how we experience life.

For example, you may have broken your leg. How you interpret the meaning of this event is your choice. You could see it as a terrible misfortune that means you are missing out on work, or you could see it as a way to catch up on all the Netflix series you have been meaning to watch, or an opportunity to relax at home with your favourite book. If you choose to see the event negatively, you are more likely to feel bad about your circumstances while the opposite is also true.

This book places the responsibility of how you choose to interpret events and situations in your life in your own hands, while at the same time guiding you towards finding what is helpful for you.

Practical

My approach is practical because it puts ideas into practice. In each session, I shall present you with:

1. An explanation of the session's content so you can consciously align with it. By understanding what needs to be done differently, you choose to collaborate with the process and set the intention of conditioning your mind in a healthy, helpful, and positive way.

2. Hypnotic audio sessions that affect positive change at the subconscious level, bypassing the conscious mind, and therefore allowing for the effortless creation of a helpful mindset.

3. Homework that involves both reflective practices and behavioural exercises. These will help you cement what you have previously learnt at the conscious and unconscious level by putting it into practice in everyday life.

Progressive and complete

The practical sessions in this book will take you on a step-by-step process that is designed to leave nothing unattended. They will not only help you overcome stage fright, but they will also show you how to thrive and excel so that you feel thrilled every time you are under the spotlight.

Is this just NLP?

To be transparent, I would like to reassure you that this book is not just NLP redressed and renamed. Before I offer you my take on NLP, I think it appropriate to provide you with some background understanding of what it is.

NLP stands for neuro-linguistic programming. It is a series of techniques developed by John Grinder and Richard Bandler in the 1970s. These men were fascinated by the idea of 'unconscious genius' epitomised by three masters in the field of psychotherapy who could affect change in patients in a highly intuitive and unconscious way. They set out to model Fritz Perls, Virginia Satir, and Milton Erickson in particular.

Friedrich Perls was a German psychotherapist who developed Gestalt therapy; Virginia Satir was the mother of Family Therapy, and Milton Erickson was an American psychologist and psychiatrist famous for his creative approach to the unconscious mind as a solution-generating apparatus. He is considered by many one of the founding fathers of hypnotherapy.

These three figures had something important in common; they were all pioneers in their field and could consistently achieve positive results treating complex clinical issues.

So, what did Richard Bandler and John Grinder do with these highly influential figures of modern psychotherapy? Bandler and Grinder's idea was that by replicating the language structure and behavioural patterns of these geniuses, they would be able to construct a language-based therapeutic model which would be capable of influencing neurological processes to achieve specific goals in life.

I find the philosophical and theoretical frameworks of NLP useful to adopt, insofar as they reflect the thoughts and methods of Perls, Satir, and Erickson. However, what I consider most useful in NLP is understanding the power of positive language structures and the use of techniques that bring about practical change.

However, I have observed in my clinical practice that these techniques are a lot more effective when used under hypnosis. This is because NLP's efficacy seems to depend on whether it is employed by highly charismatic practitioners and received by subjects who are very susceptible to suggestion with minimal input. The trouble is that only 20% of the population are somnambulists, which means they are highly susceptible to hypnosis.

The rest of the population, however, would not benefit as much from NLP exercises because their critical conscious mind gets in the way and a lot of NLP practitioners use their models 'cold' on clients by dismissing the effectiveness of the hypnotic induction.

This is a problem for most of the people with performance anxiety as they may not find it easy to relax instantly. As a result, I always use the best NLP techniques in conjunction with hypnosis, thereby enhancing their effectiveness.

Now that you know what is different about my approach, let us delve into how to make change happen fast.

PART I—

HOW TO MAKE
CHANGE HAPPEN FAST

Chapter 1

How to Make the
Most of this Book

In this chapter, I shall discuss how you can effectively use this manual to obtain maximum results.

First, I strongly encourage you to make this book yours by making notes, writing in the margins, or highlighting sections that speak to you. The more you engage with the content, the more you will get out of it. You may want to use brightly coloured pencils, write down comments, or underline passages that feel important.

The book is divided into four parts:

Part I is dedicated to understanding what underpins the sessions and practical exercises presented in part II, III, and IV. In this section, I will discuss what hypnosis is, what function the subconscious serves, the best mindset to adopt, and the options you have for using the sessions included. I will also explain how to effectively communicate to your mind to maximise the effect of the work you will do. Finally, I will offer some case studies so you can see how hypnotherapy has helped others with similar issues achieve lasting results.

In part II, III, and IV I will present you with ten transformational hypnotic sessions that will help you reduce anxiety, let go of worry and catastrophic thinking, and become more confident while performing.

Part II will help you gain a good understanding of how to deal with fear so that you can remain calmer when you feel afraid.

In part III, you will learn how to let go of the past so you can create the kind of future you dream of when it comes to performance.

In part IV, you will learn how to stop your negative thoughts and deal with self-consciousness. Then you will be ready to develop the performer mindset so you can move into a creative flow and give your best under the spotlight.

At the end of part II and IV, I will also provide you with bonus sessions covering issues such as overcoming the fear of rejection, releasing trauma, and letting go of limiting beliefs.

All sections of the book are meant to be read systematically and in sequence. Each session focuses on one issue at a time. I recommend you start from the beginning and proceed through the sections and sessions in the order they appear. However, if you strongly feel that only certain sections apply to you, I'd suggest you read the book in its entirety first so you can make an informed choice as to which sessions to complete and which ones to leave behind.

Most sessions consist of three parts:

- A short explanation of what the content is about

  This covers what we will be focussing on and why.

- The outline of a transformational hypnosis recording with a link to the corresponding audio

  Each hypnosis session starts with the 'induction'—how the hypnotic state is induced, followed by the main content.

- The homework

  These are exercises for you to engage in before moving on to the next session.

Your options

You will have the option to record each session yourself. However, to make it easier for you to benefit from the exercises, I have created a companion audio-visual online course that contains all the hypnotic audios presented in this book. If you want to take advantage of this, I have included a link to the online course in each session. The first online transformational audio is free, so you can experience what the recorded audios are like before you purchase.

If, on the other hand, you decide to create the sessions yourself, you will first need to record an induction followed by the summary of the online content which will be provided in each chapter. Be aware that this is not strictly speaking a script. Instead, it relies on you making the instructions your own by elaborating on them. You will find a full induction script in Chapter 6 along with detailed instructions on how to use it.

If you want to record the sessions yourself, I suggest you use your phone. You can download recording apps easily. Just go to Google Play on Android or your App Store on iPhone and search for 'voice recorder'.

If you already know how to hypnotise yourself, you can record silence for 10 or 15 minutes, and then record the outline of the session. However, this kind of unguided self-hypnosis practice is quite advanced and only possible after a fair bit of experience. If you want to become fluent in it, I would suggest you start by seeing a hypnotherapist who will teach you the basics. Once you feel confident, you can proceed to this more advanced technique.

If you don't know how to hypnotise yourself, go to Chapter 6 and record the hypnotic induction provided there and then add the content of the session. In addition to using the content suggested in each session, you also will have the option of recording your own suggestions or using a simple affirmation. To do this effectively, please read Bonus Session 3, where you will learn the difference between affirmations and suggestions and how to write a successful autosuggestion for maximum absorption.

Here is a summary of your options:

- **Option 1** Listen to the guided hypnotic audio included in the online course.

- **Option 2** Make up your own hypnotic audio by recording an induction followed by the content outlined in each session

- **Option 3** Make up your own hypnotic audio by leaving a blank space at the beginning of your recording, followed by the content outlined in each session.

Why so many sessions? Isn't one enough?

If you type 'overcome performance anxiety hypnotic download' on Google, you will find a plethora of audio tracks that claim to cure you of any given issue in one session. I would caution you against trusting any hypnotherapist who suggests one session is enough to 'fix' all your problems.

Although some of the downloads you will find online can be very effective, their quality varies greatly. Also, consider that it is highly unlikely one single half-hour recording will solve any complex problem in one go. Although one hypnotic recording may deal with *one part* of the issue, it most likely will leave the rest untreated.

Anyone suggesting a single download is enough, probably relies heavily on the power of positive expectation and will only be able to help you superficially. The download may be able to remove your symptoms, but if the cause of the issue is not properly treated, the problem will come back in a different form.

Therefore, in this book, I will present you with not one, but ten hypnotic sessions, timed and structured to ensure that you receive the most comprehensive course on overcoming performance anxiety available anywhere.

What to do before your session:

- Make sure you are in a quiet place where nothing can distract you. Switch off the phone and turn off your notifications. Put a sign on the door, so your kids or partner do not interrupt you. Be in a comfortable position so you can fully participate in any of the exercises and hypnosis tracks that are part of the session.

- Don't listen to the audio tracks in the bath or while driving.

- Stretch your muscles before listening to the hypnotic audio. Stretching loosens the muscles and tendons, allowing you to sit or lie more comfortably. Additionally, stretching starts the process of "going inward" and brings added focus to the body.

- Take one deep breath. Breathing deeply slows down the heart rate and relaxes the muscles to help ensure a comfortable experience during any guided exercises that will happen during the session.

- Sit on a chair with your feet on the floor and your hands not touching. Alternatively, you can lie down with your legs uncrossed and your hands not touching. If you are accustomed to meditation, you can sit on your meditation cushion. It is a good idea to always maintain the same position when going into hypnosis so your body associates the position with hypnosis and will respond more quickly each time.

How often should you listen to the recordings?

If you want change to happen fast, you need to commit. Unless otherwise specified, listen to each transformational hypnotic audio every day for at least seven days. Repetition is essential and plays a massive role in making the audio stick. Keep on listening to the sessions until you feel you have thoroughly absorbed the content.

If you wanted to become an Olympic Athlete, you would need to train every day. You couldn't just train once and then say: "It didn't work! I give up!" That would be ridiculous, right? You are about to undertake serious mental training. Like physical training, hypnosis takes practice, commitment, and repetition.

It helps to have a routine that you associate with listening to the recordings. Ideally, you could listen to them before going to bed or as soon as you wake up. Whether you listen to them or record your own, if you want *real results,* keep in mind the *hypnotic audios are not optional, but rather essential* to success.

Once the content has become part of your subconscious mind, it will be time to put these ideas into practice. This is when the 'homework' comes into play.

The homework

The homework presented in each session involves practical exercises and short assignments that will help give life to the content learned through hypnosis. By doing the homework, you are strengthening your learning with actual experience. Remember that the more you put into this process, the more you will get out of it.

In the next chapter, I shall suggest what mindset to adopt to make sure you go through the program smoothly and achieve the results you deserve.

Chapter 2

The Mindset for Success

In this chapter, I shall suggest what kind of attitude will give you the best results so you can successfully go through the program and easily achieve your performance goals.

The right mindset for success

If you want to succeed in overcoming your difficulties around performing, you need to have the right attitude. To do so, I would suggest you adopt the following mindset:

- Challenge the myth that others can rescue you; only you can save yourself.

- Take responsibility for change.

- Be convinced that you really have a choice.

Although this book shall be your trustworthy guide every step of the way, ultimately, it is you who must do the work. If you expect a quick fix, you will be disappointed. But if you put in the work and take responsibility for your success, you will make huge progress quicker than you anticipate. You need to believe in your capacity to do this, because doubt is self-sabotage.

Here's a metaphor I often use to describe the process of taking control:

Imagine you are an adult living in a house ruled by undisciplined kids. If you do not believe you are the one in charge, the kids will do whatever they want to—run amok, and make a mess of things. The first step in getting them to recognise your authority is to believe you are in control and act accordingly. It might take a while to educate the kids on this new status quo, but over time, firm boundaries and commitment will do the trick.

Your thoughts are a little bit like those unruly children. You need to first decide you are going to be the rightful master of the house, and then consistently and patiently practice your authority by focusing on the thoughts you want to stimulate. As you repetitively engage in the hypnotic sessions, your mind will become your best friend rather than your enemy, and you will be truly in charge of a harmonious and peaceful household.

In terms of this course, here are some principles I would urge you to abide by so you can be fully in charge of your success.

I am the coach and you are the expert on you

Remember that you—not I—are the expert on you. I am a coach; not a guru, a sage, or a superior being with limitless knowledge about how to be happy and successful.

I am not here to fix you. You are already okay! I am only here to help you find your own answers and generate your own perfect solutions so you can be the best performer you can be. This course is not about being passive or placid, and the measure of your success is equal to your capacity to actively engage in the process.

Imagine you wanted to build a wardrobe in your house, but you'd never done it before. You could attempt to do it on your own and you may succeed, but it would probably involve many mistakes, a few headaches, some money wasted, and a quite a bit of time. If, on the other hand, you asked someone who had done it before to tell you what materials to get, how to go about building it, and what mistakes to watch out for, it would end up being faster, easier, and probably a more enjoyable project.

I am that person for you. You still need to do the work yourself, but by the end of it, you get to feel good about yourself having learnt a bunch of new skills and knowing you can use them again for other projects.

When you are motivated to change and you have positive expectations, you are already half-way there. View the whole process you are embarking on as a project you are undertaking with the help of a supervising expert who has done it all before.

Focus on what you want, not what you don't want

Imagine you are planning a trip. You first need to think of where you are going. What is your destination? Maybe you want to go to Paris. If so, it makes sense to focus on going to Paris, rather than spending all your time thinking about the fact that you don't want to go to Moscow! If you were a skier and wanted to get down the slope during a slalom, it would make sense for you pay attention to the route, not the poles on the way. So, focus on the destination you have chosen, not the obstacles; pay attention to the solution, not the problem; think of what you want, not what you don't want.

Trust the process

It's night and you are in a car. Your headlights are on, but you can only see a few meters ahead. You are going quite fast, but you trust that all you need to see is only what is in front of you. There is no way for you to know what the road is going to be like in one, two, or ten kilometres. You just trust you will deal with it when you get there.

This is the attitude that is going to help you the most while working through this book. Don't try to figure it all out in advance. Just trust that all you need to know is the next step, and then the next, and the next. All shall be revealed in time. Your car will take you there. You don't need to know *how*. You just need to pay full attention to the present moment.

Expect success

The subconscious is a goal-striving mechanism that is image based and emotion driven. This means that when using hypnosis, we want to use words that are highly evocative of strong, positive emotions and avoid analytical reasoning. The subconscious will follow your commands, provided you consciously approve of them. This ensures that no involuntary actions are possible.

The success formula for harnessing the power of our subconscious is to use the imagination in conjunction with positive emotion and expectation. In other words, you need to imagine what you want; imagine success, and expect it. Picture what it would feel like to have success already in your life and fill in the details until you are really connected to the emotions that would emerge when your dream is a reality. Believe success is not just possible, but a certainty. You cannot fail until you quit, so don't give up until you succeed!

Don't test hypnosis

If you try to test the effectiveness of hypnosis, you are effectively giving yourself a suggestion that it may fail to work. Your subconscious will take this cue and produce the very results you fear.

When you are in doubt or indulge in anxious thoughts about results, you are expressing a pattern of your fear, of powerful negative expectations which will tend to be realised. If you indulge in thoughts of resistance, you are once again giving yourself the suggestion that you are resistant, and of course, your subconscious will play up to your suggestion until you give yourself a strong and definite counter suggestion.

While it is normal to be doubtful or scared at times, indulging in these patterns causes trouble. You can decide how much energy and attention you give these thoughts. You can't stop a bird from flying over your head, but you don't have to build it a nest! So, do yourself a favour and express confidence in the power of your subconscious and in the power of hypnosis. Positive expectation, anticipating positive results, getting excited about them, and trusting the process are good ways to help hypnotherapy work for you.

Plan, engage, and commit

Be honest with yourself about your progress. It's okay to take your time with this course and to do it at your own pace. Do not put yourself under too much pressure to finish it quickly, but also commit to a specific amount of weekly practice. Once you know what is reasonable given your other commitments, you will have a general timeframe by which you will have completed the course. Put that date on your calendar and plan your sessions accordingly. Mark the sessions as you complete them. This way, you will always know where you are in the process.

Surrender to each stage of the journey

Surrendering to the present is essential if we want to be able to move forward. Accepting where you are at during each stage of the journey, accepting your situation and the way you feel about it, is a stepping stone to creating a better future. Trying to avoid what is happening right now by focusing on the past, what should be, or what you don't want, means that you are wasting energy that could be better used in becoming open to the possibilities for change inherent in what you are experiencing in the present moment.

Let go of judgement

With judgement of ourselves and others comes shame and blame, which will only keep you stuck in the negative. The invitation here is to become aware of when you become caught up in judgement, so you can focus instead on what is helpful.

Take responsibility to empower yourself

It is important that you become honest and accountable to yourself and acknowledge your flawed thinking. Do you prefer complaining about problems rather than looking for solutions? Do you frequently blame other people for what is not working in your life, or do you face up to what needs changing? Do you complain that life isn't fair or can you acknowledge your own influence in creating situations?

Taking responsibility is not about self-blame. It is about realising that nobody is going to save you or give you the answers you seek. It is about moving away from helplessness and victim mentality. It is shifting away from the mindset that life is something that happens *to you* and towards being in charge of your own reality, with the power to create and reinvent yourself. Use this book to help you do exactly that.

Be willing to introspect and engage with the process of inner discovery

I sometimes joke that my clients are only allowed one 'I don't know' per session. If you find yourself saying it after a question I pose to you, I encourage you to go beyond it. Pause and look deeper within. Take a breath and listen. Be patient and as you look within, you will discover what is behind the 'I don't know' answer.

Be accountable for keeping your own agreements and carrying out the set-out tasks

You are your word. You are the measure for how much you show up. Your commitment is the measure of your success. Commitment means giving a task 100%. When engaging in homework tasks, it is important to be aware of your expectations. As an active participant, you are invited to either agree or disagree with a suggested task or to re-negotiate a task with yourself in a way that fits your needs.

Be willing to stay with the discomfort and challenge yourself

Discomfort is sometimes necessary to achieve goals. Challenges are opportunities for growth. Problems contain an inner gift that allows us to go beyond what we thought was possible. Stepping out of your comfort zone is necessary to move towards your dreams. When you relish pushing yourself forward while at the same time remembering you can manifest your goals step-by-step, you ensure you will achieve them without overwhelm.

Reward yourself

Every time you stick to the program, give yourself a reward. For example, you could put a coin in a jar for each session you have completed. At the end of the program, you could use the money to treat yourself with a gift! Every time you stray, just get back in line. Starve distractions and create a routine so you make it easy for yourself to listen to the audio recordings. For example, you could listen to the sessions at the same time every day. Alternatively, you could set a reminder on your phone so that you remember to do so every day.

Motivate yourself by keeping your benefits in mind

Always keep in mind the benefits you are going to experience from engaging fully in the process. Your mental health and wellbeing are at stake! If I told you I would give you a million dollars if you did a hundred star jumps a day for twenty days, wouldn't you make sure you'd remember to do it? Well, this is easier than doing star jumps. And the reward is your own happiness and life satisfaction. How much is that worth to you?

If you find it easier to connect to your negative motivation, think of the price you are going to pay for staying where you are. Is that worth your comfort? Give this process all you've got and you shall reap your rewards a thousand-fold.

Celebrate mistakes

Remember to always celebrate mistakes. They are the only way to learn. If you were born already perfect, all-knowing, and doing everything right, what would there be left to do?

A baby is not born knowing how to talk, walk, or feed herself. She must try and will get it wrong many times. Does she give up? No! She has no concept of mistakes. She is just here to explore and learn. See if you can take on the attitude of that baby. If you have children, you can learn a lot from them!

I'm very glad that you've come to this point in your life where you feel you are ready to begin to make the changes that you want to make. This is the beginning of a wonderful process in which you will discover the true power of your mind and it is exciting for me to be part of it.

In this chapter, I have explained the mindset that is best adopted to make the most of the sessions in part II, III, and IV of this book.

In the next chapter, I will describe the six fundamental mind hacks you need to be aware of to effectively communicate with your mind so you can achieve the results you desire and enjoy lasting success in the process of inner transformation.

Chapter 3

The Six Fundamental
Mind Hacks for Achieving
Lasting Success

When you understand how to communicate effectively with your mind, you will be able to get the most benefit out of the sessions because you will know how to use hypnosis to influence it. To do so, you need to know how to make your subconscious do what you want it to do, *not what you don't.*

Partly borrowed and adapted from Marisa Peer's[2] framework, here is my method for hacking your mind so it becomes your best friend rather than your worst enemy.

HACK 1—Your mind does what it thinks you want it to

From the moment you come into this world, your subconscious has one job: to keep you alive for as long as possible. It does that by taking you away from pain and moving you towards pleasure.

It is easy for your mind to know what gives you physical pain, but how about psychological pain? After all, an event could be pleasurable for some and painful for others. Some people love to jump off planes with a parachute. For others, that would be the picture of hell.

---

[2] Marisa Peer has written books on confidence, self-esteem, and fertility, and I would recommend her framework if you're interested in knowing more about how the mind works.

To know what is psychologically painful or pleasurable to you, your subconscious gathers information by listening to what you say to yourself and noticing the positive or negative meaning you assign to events.

Once your mind knows what you think is good or bad for you, it will transform that into a belief that will inform your future actions. So, if you think snakes are fun, you will become excited by the prospect of handling pythons. If, on the other hand, you tell yourself that talking to a stranger is hell, then your mind will most probably make sure you avoid all social situations so that you are not in danger of suffering.

HACK 2—Your mind responds to only two things

Your subconscious is always listening, and it responds to only two things:

- *The words you say to yourself (inside your own head and aloud)*

- *The pictures you create in your mind.*

The words you say to yourself automatically produce pictures in your head.

Since your mind does not distinguish between what you imagine and what you experience, it responds to the pictures you imagine as if they were real.

Your words are powerful. Language shapes our perception. People who speak different languages will especially know what I am talking about. If you don't have a word for something, it might as well not exist. Naming something gives it power, because the brain immediately creates pictures when we use 'picture words' such as nouns.

The implication of this is massive. How many times have you been told not to do something and ended up doing that very thing? If you have kids, you will know that the worst thing you can tell them is not to touch an object, because now, they immediately want to touch it. The fact is trying *not to do* something is the best way to assure we continue doing it.

Here's an example. Try not to think of a red bus. Just don't think of a red bus. Do anything you like, but don't think of a red bus. What are you thinking about?

So, negative language will produce the very result you fear. Why? Because when we formulate thoughts, we immediately associate images, sounds, and sensations to create an idea in our minds of the objects and states described in the thoughts. But words such as "don't" or "not" have no actual content—they are not 'picture words'; they only make sense when paired with an object or state they are trying to negate.

In other words, a red bus is a real thing we can imagine. The word "not" is nothing in and of itself and makes sense only as far as it is paired with *something else* which we will immediately imagine. So, signs such as "don't forget to lock the door" might as well be translated in our brain as "lock the door". This is super important for trying to condition ourselves, because if we feed our attention with what we don't want, we will get exactly that.

When you remind yourself of what you don't want, your mind doesn't register the negatives, and moves you towards the very things you don't want. When you spend all your time saying to yourself, "I hate performing", "Giving presentations is hell", "I am going to forget what I am saying", "I am going to make a fool of myself", "My throat is going to dry up", "Interviews are torture", "I am terrified", "I'd rather do anything else", "I am terrible at speaking in public", and so on, your mind is listening—its job is to keep you away from pain, remember? So, when it hears your words, it thinks, "Torture? Hell? Hate?" it responds with, "I'd better get you out of it then! Perhaps I'll give you a panic attack, the flu, a migraine, or I'll make you lose your voice!"

I used to endlessly worry that I would forget parts of my songs while performing. During a concert, I would repeat to myself, "Oh, God! What if I forgot the lyrics? What if I forgot the chords? That would be terrible! I bet I'll forget them at exactly the wrong moment". Although I have been performing the same songs for years and I know them like the back of my hand, as soon as I thought those words, my mind would be listening and bang, the lyrics would vanish.

Once I finally realised I was telling my subconscious to produce the very result I feared, I turned my inner dialogue around. I began to say, "I remember the words of my songs perfectly. My memory is flawless. My voice knows what to do. It all just flows out of me automatically"… and—Bang! —I haven't had a problem ever since.

Your mind forms a blueprint based entirely on the words you use and the pictures those words make, and your body matches that blueprint. The moral of the story is this: be very careful what you say to yourself. Avoid using negation. Imagine what you want!

HACK 3—Emotion trumps logic

Your thoughts control your feelings, your feelings control your actions, and your actions influence events. How you interpret these events will influence your thinking and the loop will go on.

Once you have said something negative to yourself such as, "I am terrified of speaking in front of an audience" or "I always botch up my interviews", this thought will produce a negative emotion in you. The latter will in turn produce a physical reaction, such as a nervous stomach, shaky hands, or a trembling voice. You cannot control this chain of events because it's an automatic response.

So, if you want to change how you behave, you need to change your feelings, and to change your feelings, you need to *change your thinking first*. You may have noticed thoughts sometimes come automatically to you, out of habit. If you have spent your entire life telling yourself that you are a terrible speaker, that is the first thought you'll have when asked to give a speech.

Once you become aware of that thought, you have a choice. You can indulge it, or you can dismiss it. You can feed it and repeat it and believe it, or you can starve it of attention, ridicule it, doubt it, and flip it over to its opposite. Which one will you do?

HACK 4—Repetition is the key to changing your beliefs

If you repeat something to yourself long enough, your mind will believe it. Your subconscious does not care whether what you tell it is true or false, good or bad, healthy or unhealthy.

Your mind accepts whatever you tell it repetitively as true. This is even more relevant in hypnosis, because you bypass the conscious critical factor.

Remember, whatever you focus on expands. Whatever you focus on, you get more of. The plant you feed is the one that grows. The plant that you starve is the one that dies.

HACK 5—What you expect tends to be realised

Remember that what you expect is almost always realised. What happens in the outer world is a reflection of what is happening in your inner world. As I said before: you don't see reality as it is, but as *you are*. Your thoughts are a blueprint that your mind and body work together to meet.

So, be careful to always expect the best and accept the rest. Although you cannot influence what others do, you can influence how you interpret and respond to events.

If you go to a meeting expecting everybody to hate you, you will probably behave in such an awkward and insecure way that people will not like you much. But since outer reality is a mirror of your inner reality, you have no better way of trying to influence other people's response to you than expecting them to like you because you like yourself.

When you say to yourself that you are liked and accepted, you will behave in a more friendly way and the right people will respond positively. If they don't you also have a choice. You can see it as a disaster and proof that you are worthless, or you can see it as a blessing; they are not your tribe. Now you know who your real friends are.

So, expect the ideal outcome of any situation. Put in your best effort and trust that is all you can do. This way you will be likely to influence your outcome with a good attitude and even if you do not obtain the result you anticipated, you are more likely to take it well and not unreasonably conclude that it's all your fault.

HACK 6—Your mind loves what is familiar and rejects what is unfamiliar.

Your mind loves familiarity because it makes evolutionary sense. If something is familiar, it is something you already know. So, it is more likely that you know how to deal with it if things go wrong.

Your subconscious loves what it already knows because it makes it feel safe. But of course, if you stay 'safe' in your comfort zone, you will never grow. And if your comfort zone is full of negative habits, you can end up being safe in hell. To hack your mind, you need to make the unfamiliar familiar and the familiar unfamiliar.

If, for example, you constantly put yourself down whenever you make a mistake, that will become very familiar to you, and as such it will feel natural. If I then suggested you replaced that negative habit with a practice of self-encouragement, you may find the new behaviour very unfamiliar. But by consciously deciding to start praising yourself when you do well and to be more compassionate and gentler when you don't, you will begin to feel better and you will achieve better results.

The trick is to decide to make the familiar behaviour less familiar by repeatedly replacing it with a more helpful behaviour. For example, if you practiced replacing self-criticism with a willingness to forgive yourself and a decision to learn from your mistakes, over time, it would become more natural to be gentle with yourself and the self-criticism would stop.

Begin by noticing what your negative self-talk is saying. How does it relate to the above? To kickstart change, we need to recognise our go-to negative beliefs and flip them over to their respective opposite. In Audio Session 2, I will show you how to do this in detail and in Bonus Session 3, I will outline how to create auto suggestions and affirmations to develop better beliefs.

How to apply these hacks

The best thing you can do to help yourself overcome performance anxiety is to always keep the above rules in mind. To overcome negative beliefs, self-criticism, and self-doubt, is to improve your self-esteem. When your self-esteem goes up, so does your performance. So, pay attention to your self-talk. What language are you using? What are you expecting? What are you focusing on?

When you notice negative expectations and negative inner dialogue, stop, and take a breath. Are these beliefs serving you or disempowering you? What are you communicating to your mind? Is this what you want?

Remember that most problems in life stem from adopting the following negative core beliefs:

- you are not good enough.

- you don't belong.

- you can't have what you want.

It's a good idea to begin by flipping these over to their opposite:

- I am good enough.

- I belong.

- I can have what I want.

I would suggest you include these fundamental positive core beliefs in your self-hypnosis suggestions. To find out how to do that, read Bonus Session 3.

In this chapter, I have shown you the fundamental ways in which you can influence your mind.

In the next chapter, I will show you how hypnosis can help you achieve your performance goals.

Chapter 4

Hypnosis Demystified

In this chapter, I will explain what hypnosis is, what to expect during a session, and I will offer answers to some common questions about what hypnosis can and cannot do.

What is hypnosis?

Hypnotherapists have defined hypnosis in many ways. Some people believe it is a state, some think it is not. I do not wish to delve into this debate here, because I find it irrelevant for our purposes, but if you are interested in learning more about it, I recommend you read Adam Eason's book, *The Science of Self-Hypnosis*.

Here is my practical working definition: hypnosis is a skill that allows us to create a state of focussed awareness. It is a process where inner focus, concentration and often, but not always, relaxation, are predominant. This process or state allows us to access the subconscious so we can learn new patterns of thought and behaviour.

Hypnosis as a "state" feels similar to both the hypnagogic and hypnopompic stages of falling asleep and waking up from sleep. The hypnagogic state occurs when we are about to fall asleep and we are aware of the room around us, but we pay it no heed. The hypnopompic state occurs when we have just woken up, but our eyes are closed and we are not fully awake.

Lucid dreaming also resembles hypnosis in that during this state, we can direct our dreams via our conscious mind and in hypnosis, the hypnotist aids us in directing our subconscious to create dream-like scenarios. However, during hypnosis, we are not dreaming as such.

Hypnosis is also similar to meditation, but it differs from it in the way it is induced and in what it is used for. Hypnosis could be called 'directed daydreaming' where the hypnotherapist guides you through unknown territories by offering you a map and a set of instructions. Nevertheless, you as the traveller are in control.

No-one can force you into hypnosis if you don't want to be hypnotised—and for this reason, all hypnosis is essentially self-hypnosis. It is your opportunity to discover the power of your own imagination, and you remain in total control of your own openness to this.

Hypnotic 'trances' happen naturally every day without you even realising it, for example, when you are driving a car and you suddenly realise you don't know how you arrived at your destination. Or when you are reading a book and suddenly you turn the page and have no idea what you've been reading. Or when you are going from the kitchen to the bedroom to fetch something and when you get there, you can't remember why you went there. All these times, you were lost in an unconscious daydream.

You are also in a 'trance' when you are deeply absorbed in an activity; for example, when you've been engrossed in a movie or video game and you don't even notice your partner coming into the room and asking you a question. Or perhaps you are practicing a song you really like, and forget to eat. Or you are a character in a show and suddenly it's all over and you don't remember much about what you said. Or you may have your gaze fixed on nothing in particular until someone waves their hand in front of your eyes and asks, "Hello? Are you there?"

Other examples of being in a natural trance are when you are experiencing an intense emotion, such as being in shock when someone shouts at you during an argument, or feeling intense happiness when in love. Children are almost always in a trance, especially when they play. The only difference between these naturally occurring states and a hypnotic trance is that during hypnosis the 'trance' is voluntarily induced and used for a specific purpose. It is the way we use it that really matters here.

When we are hypnotised, we are more suggestible and able to learn because the conscious mind is bypassed. The latter's job is to filter information and decide what is accepted into your system and what is not. By bypassing the conscious mind, you become able to update any erroneous unconscious 'programs' about your experiences and interpretations of the world stored in your subconscious.

Some people are better at hypnosis than others, because it is a skill, and as such, like a muscle, it becomes stronger with use. The hypnotic mindset will greatly help you become highly skilled in a relatively short period of time. According to Theodore Barber[3], the most important thing is to recognise that hypnotic responses are attributed to you, not to the hypnotist. The hypnotic mindset[4] can be summarised as follows:

- You expect hypnosis to happen.

- You recognise the induction as a cue to become hypnotised.

- You choose to see suggestions as an opportunity—an array of possibilities that are open to you, rather than a threat.

- You realise you are in control and you are confident you can enter hypnosis (but you don't try too hard, either).

- You commit to wait for your body to respond. You are involved in the process; this is not just something the hypnotist does to you.

- You are aware of what you are doing. You think about your experience, and you become the observer.

---

[3] Theodore X Barber was an American psychologist who wrote among others: Hypnosis: A Scientific Approach (1969)

Biofeedback and Self-Control (1971)

Hypnosis, Imagination, and Human Potentialities (1974)

Advances in Altered States of Consciousness & Human Potentialities (1976)

[4] For more detailed explanations of the hypnotic mindset refer to "The Science of Self-Hypnosis" by Adam Eason p32-34

How does hypnosis feel?

Hypnosis is not a state of unconsciousness, but rather a state of heightened awareness. Therefore, it's nothing like being hit in the head and passing out! During hypnosis, you are aware of everything that is happening around you. You are simply focused on one idea at a time, or at least, that is what you are aiming for.

Although you may become absorbed in that idea and forget where you are generally, you will feel too relaxed and comfortable to want to think about it. Hypnosis is often coupled with extreme relaxation, but this is not always necessary.

The feeling of being 'under' hypnosis often entails a sense of physical relaxation. Your muscles may feel pleasantly relaxed. However, the degree of relaxation changes from one hypnotic experience to another. Over time and with practice, it will become easier to experience deep relaxation.

When the body relaxes, so does the mind, and it is common to feel like sounds around you do not really bother you. In a way, it's like the feeling of falling asleep with a TV running somewhere faintly in the background, or watching yourself sleep in your mind's eye.

Of course, sounds could be interpreted as distracting or annoying, but that only depends on your attitude! The choice is yours. You can continue to think your thoughts, but it is up to you how much attention you pay to them. The objective is to watch yourself think and train your attention to focus on what is beneficial to you.

Many people are not sure whether they have been hypnotised or not. This is because of their expectations.

If you have watched a lot of stage hypnosis shows, you would have seen people who seem to be under the hypnotist's spell and have no will of their own. It's important to remember that stage hypnosis is a show. The audience is made of people who have paid for tickets and expect unusual things to happen. The stage hypnotist goes through compliance procedures before calling receptive subjects onto the stage. The illusion is built around the participants not wanting to do the things that they are told to do, but during hypnosis, their conscious inhibitions are sidestepped and this gives them a chance to let loose. Sounds like a good idea if you want to become a performer yourself, right?

As a result of watching these shows, you may be expecting hypnosis to feel like sleep or unconsciousness. Although it is possible you may fall asleep while under hypnosis, this does not generally happen. One clue to know whether you have been hypnotised or not, is to ask yourself how much time you think has passed since you started your session. Just like during sleep, time seems to pass more quickly during hypnosis than it normally does. Usually, hypnotised people are surprised to find that more time has elapsed since the beginning of their session than previously anticipated.

During the hypnotic session, you retain all control. You could choose to reject all suggestions, but you'd be wasting your time. You could try to objectively test its effectiveness, but you'd be running the risk of creating a self-fulfilling prophecy and getting the negative results you expect. You'll have to trust me on this: self-hypnosis works.

You can also 'wake up' at any time during hypnosis. Nobody has ever been trapped in a hypnotic state and any sensationalist story you may have heard to that effect, is completely unfounded. Sometimes, people enjoy being hypnotised so much that they refuse to awaken at the hypnotist's command. When this happens, they will eventually fall asleep and wake up when they are ready. Once again, this shows you that you are ultimately the one in control of the whole process.

There are different depths of hypnosis, generally classified as light, medium, and deep. As a beginner, you may only go as far as a 'light trance' until you become more used to the experience. This is enough for our purposes. It is likely you will fluctuate between light and deeper states of relaxation and awareness during each session, and it is important to not become too hung up on this as you will experience the same benefits, regardless of the depth of hypnosis.

If, during the hypnotic sessions, you find you have thoughts such as 'Am I really hypnotised?' or 'Am I deep enough?' or 'Is this really working?' remember that is your conscious mind thinking. You can make a choice to ignore these thoughts and trust that your subconscious knows what to do if you let those questions go for the moment.

As you hear my voice, it's enough to have the *intention* to listen and to absorb the beneficial ideas I'm suggesting. It doesn't matter whether you are consciously listening or not, although if you are concentrating on something irrelevant to the session, this is likely to negatively influence the outcome. Your unconscious mind will absorb anything it intends to absorb, and you can trust it to do its work.

Some of the most common sensations you may experience during a session are:

- Your legs and your arms may feel heavier or lighter than normal.

- You may feel a sensation similar to floating or sinking into the floor.

- You may think a part of your body is in a different position from where it really is.

- You may not feel some parts of your body at all.

- You may see images or colours in your mind.

- You may wake up feeling revitalised and calm, as if you've had a power nap.

During the sessions, I will ask you to imagine objects or scenarios. When I do, be aware that I do not expect you to have a hallucination or a dream. If you can have a clear visual image, it's fantastic, but you don't have to be seeing an actual picture. All that is required is that you imagine the place or situation I suggest—you sense it, you think about it, you feel it, you know it or you simply pretend that you are there as much as you can.

The best way to make use of hypnosis, is to allow whatever happens to happen without trying to grasp what you think should or shouldn't happen. Let it happen anyway. In the process of doing that, you will learn to be the master of your mind. You will no longer be at the mercy of your own thoughts; you will be the one who decides what to pay more or less attention to.

Common misconceptions about hypnosis

Hypnotism is not magic and although no harm has ever come to anyone because of hypnotherapy, it is common for the general public to have fantastical ideas about what it can do.

It is natural to resist what we do not understand. However, it is much more dangerous to not understand the power of hypnosis. This power does not stem from the hypnotist, but from your own subconscious mind, and if you do not channel it, it can control you. Psychosomatic illnesses are the result of this uncontrolled power working against you when you could easily use it to your advantage.

Fear of hypnosis is gradually being replaced by acceptance. This is mainly due to evidence-based studies and research demonstrating its beneficial effects. This in turn, has led the medical profession to finally accept it as a valuable therapy. Some psychiatrists and psychotherapists are now beginning to supplement psychotherapy with hypnotherapy, producing results previously obtained in more than double the time.

"Hypnobirthing" has been used countless times to help women give birth without epidurals and there are well-documented cases of entire operations being conducted without general anaesthetic by simply using hypnosis.

Can hypnosis make you do something you don't want to do?

If I could use hypnosis to make people do my bidding, would I waste my time writing this book or seeing clients? Would I not be wiser to just go to my bank manager and ask him to give me all his money and then give him amnesia?

Remember that to be hypnotised, you need to want to. The only people who cannot be hypnotised are people who don't want to be, or people who cannot concentrate enough, such as people with dementia or very young children.

Everyone else can be hypnotised, even people that are convinced they cannot relax. All you need is an open mind, the willingness to have progressive and motivated thoughts about the process, the positive expectation that it will work for you, and the commitment to follow the procedure so that the session can help you make the changes you want and deserve.

In this chapter, I gave a brief overview of hypnosis and clarified some common misconceptions around it. In the next chapter, I shall discuss the difference between the conscious, subconscious, and unconscious mind, why the subconscious is so powerful, and how to access it effectively.

Chapter 5

The Subconscious Explained

The conscious, subconscious, and unconscious mind

Some people think that hypnosis involves being unconscious. This isn't true—not much can be achieved when you're fully unconscious! Hypnosis is about developing deeper awareness.

Let's be clear: the conscious mind is really another way to describe conscious awareness. When we ask ourselves questions such as, 'What am I going to have for dinner?', 'What should I do today?' we are consciously analysing events and feelings and making decisions about them.

When, on the other hand, I talk about 'the unconscious' mind, I don't mean that there is a place in the brain where the unconscious resides. Instead, I am using the word 'unconscious' as a metaphor signifying all the processes that happen underneath the surface of conscious awareness. These processes remain unconscious, such as breathing, cell regeneration, blood circulation, and movement coordination.

In the same way, when I talk about the 'subconscious mind' I also don't mean that there is such a 'thing' somewhere in the brain. What I am really referring to is any process that you are not 'yet' aware of. You can always dredge up the information residing under your conscious awareness by an act of the will.

For example, you may not be constantly aware of all the phone numbers you have memorised, but when required, you can recall the number you want—provided you focus your attention and you calmly and patiently wait for the answer. Note that this needs to be done in a relaxed frame of mind, or the conscious mind will interfere and stop the automatic process from working seamlessly.

The subconscious mind is the part of us where dreams, feelings, memories, attitudes, and behaviours are created and stored and where they can be changed. All the wonders our bodies perform every day depend on unconscious knowledge. Think of how many chemical, physiological, and mechanical series of commands and interactions are involved in walking alone.

Although as a baby, you had to consciously learn how to stand and walk on your two legs, once you learnt how, your unconscious took over and started doing it automatically without you having to think about it. Your subconscious mind makes adjustments that no machine could make. It keeps your body healthy and heals your wounds without you having to tell it how.

Medicines are of course useful, but all they are doing is setting up a chemical reaction to which the subconscious healing 'intelligence' reacts. Once obstacles are removed by surgical or mechanical interventions, we can use purely mental methods to arouse this self-healing power and use it to heal our ailments faster and more effectively. This does not mean that other therapies are not useful, but hypnosis is a practical and safe way to use our mental curative force to help ourselves become healthy and stay so for longer.

Before you start considering making changes in your subconscious mind, it is necessary for you to explore and understand its nature. Here is a list of its major functions as understood by Charles Tebbetts[5]

The functions of the subconscious

1) It is where our emotions reside.

Every act we ponder is the result of a choice that most often happens without full awareness. When confronted with a choice we always do the thing we most want to do subconsciously. In the presence of conflict, our

---

[5] Self-Hypnosis and other mind-expanding techniques - Charles Tebbetts p13-19

subconscious motives will always win over the conscious ones and this accounts for subconscious dominance over conscious will. Since emotions determine how strong our desires will be and since the latter determine what action we will take, we are at the mercy of our subconscious, unless we learn to guide it.

The subconscious is dominated by emotions. While we tend to think analytically when the conscious mind dominates our awareness, we understand and see things in a very different way in subconscious mode. Mostly, we tend to colour our thoughts with the emotions that are attached to the perceptions we have of ourselves and the world.

Emotions such as fear—or its opposite, trust—help direct our thoughts and create positive or negative attitudes which affect our lives. In many cases, this can mean the difference between success and failure.

Subconscious reasoning works differently from analytical reasoning. The former is restricted to deduction, which means that it draws every logical conclusion from a given premise. This deductive process, however, will elaborate conclusions from false premises just as logically as it will from true ones.

This is how misconceptions are created, since the correctness of a deduction depends solely on whether the initial premise is correct, regardless of how logical the deduction may be. Consequently, whatever the subconscious is told, it will believe.

The conscious mind functions as a filter for the subconscious and decides which premises are correct and which aren't, but it only starts to develop in adolescence. This explains why most beliefs that are deeply rooted in adults are a result of childhood suggestions involuntarily given by parents and friends.

If such beliefs go unquestioned, they will shape the self-understanding of the future adult, whether he or she likes it, or not. Such subconscious beliefs can therefore cure you or kill you, depending on whether they are based on positive and true premises or on negative and false ones.

Luckily, with the use of hypnosis, a revision of destructive misconceptions is possible and can make the difference between a lifetime of slavery to negative emotions and a lifetime of freedom to choose one's own beliefs.

2) *It's the RAM of your mind.*

Because subconsciousness is the seat of memory and emotions, it keeps an emotional record of all our experiences. This does not mean that it acts like a film camera, capturing what has happened to us in a realistic fashion. Instead, it behaves more like a still camera with a filter, as your memory of an event will be coloured by how you feel about it.

Whatever affects our senses, will leave a subconscious impression, and when the right conditions are provided, details of our personal past may be recalled. The secret of a good memory is not really a matter of retaining impressions, but of making clear ones, relating them properly together and bringing them to the surface of consciousness when needed. Usually, interference in this three-fold process accounts for difficulty in remembering.

3) *It governs our habits.*

The subconscious controls not only your negative habits, such as smoking or biting nails, but also more automatic activities such as driving a car, getting dressed, or playing tennis. This means that once you have learned how to perform such actions, you no longer have to direct them with your conscious mind. Your subconscious takes over and usually does a better job of it, as you'd discover if you tried to consciously think of which leg to move while you're running down the stairs.

The best way to get rid of a negative habit is to replace it with a positive one. This is done by first understanding what triggers it and then becoming aware of the function it serves. Once those factors are clear, we can use hypnosis to learn a different reaction to the trigger and to serve the function in a 'updated' and helpful way.

4) *It is the seat of the imagination, intuition, and dreams.*

If you think you have no imagination, think again. You are probably not aware of it but you may be using it in a way that goes against your best interests. As children, we are in touch with our imagination. Then, due to negative conditioning and painful experiences, we may become scared of using it.

I once met a woman who was told as a little girl that if she really wanted something, all she needed to do was to imagine it and she would receive it. So that's what she did. Every day, she imagined the bicycle she wanted and believed it would magically appear. Of course, it didn't, as imagination *without action* is useless.

When the bike failed to materialise, she decided she would never again imagine anything she wanted, so she could avoid disillusionment. Still, her imagination continued to work undirected, and it transformed her into a pessimist who only imagined what she feared. Since the subconscious is a goal striving mechanism, it will strive toward whatever image you present it with. If you only have images of failure and disappointment, that's what you will get. Uncontrolled negative imagination can destroy you.

If you imagine your partner to be unfaithful, you will act towards him or her in a way that will facilitate the occurrence of his or her unfaithfulness. If you imagine people hating your performance you may act in such a way that will make it more likely they will. Creative imagination on the other hand, is one of the great secrets of success.

Once you have chosen your goal, all you need to do is to formulate a clear, distinct image of the result you desire, without concerning yourself with the process. If you focus on the outcome and you work positively to achieve it, you most likely will get it.

So, if you imagine yourself as a likeable, loving, friendly person who expresses herself well on stage, you will be more likely to feel confident and you will find performing easier over time. Whether you choose to use your imagination creatively or to let it run you, the choice is yours. It can either help you achieve what you want, or it can become your worst enemy.

5) *It controls the direction of our energy.*

Imagine you are on board a ship, but the crew are out of control. The ship has been captain-less for as long as you can remember, and the crew just do what they have always done. They have an old map that directs the ship to 'failure island'. They will keep on using that old map unless the captain orders them to change course.

For you to go to 'success island' you need to take charge. Set your destination, set sail, and whenever the ship goes off course due to bad weather or unexpected sea conditions, you'll need to remind the crew of the new destination. Remember, your crew (your subconscious) are used to going to 'failure island', so they will try to get you there, but you need to remind them repeatedly that you are going to a new destination until it becomes a given.

When you try to do something new, you are going to be uncomfortable at some stage. This is because new things are by their own nature out of your comfort zone. You haven't acquired the skills needed to navigate this new territory yet. On top of that, there is always something that can go wrong which is out of your control. As humans, we try to avoid discomfort as a matter of course. We are optimised to chase pleasure and avoid pain. This means that when we feel discomfort, we will fall into an automatic habit of trying to find the easiest way out of it.

The problem with this behaviour is that the short-term benefit might also carry a hefty long-term cost. Being stuck in the present discomfort (and wanting to avoid it) and not being able to see the long-term consequences of your short-term actions is what causes the problem in the first place.

So, what do we need to do? We need to take a pause, lean into the discomfort, and understand it as a scientist would. We need to become an outside observer. What meaning are you giving to this temporary hiccup? And what are the real consequences of taking the easy way out? When you are able to properly see the long-term benefits and costs inherent in your decisions, you can make a conscious choice that takes you closer to your goal, not further away from it.

The energy that directs our behaviour cannot be stopped or shut down; it can only be directed. If its direction isn't controlled, it will be directed by chance, circumstance, or negative beliefs. Since the subconscious constantly and automatically uses this energy to proceed towards a goal, unless you set a goal for it to achieve, it will either choose one based on previously acquired beliefs, or it will proceed towards a goal someone else has suggested. If you don't give it a clear, positive direction, it will follow the 'old map' and navigate the ship towards 'bad performance', 'failure island', or some other destructive outcome.

The woman who applies for a job, but then gives up and doesn't go to the interview, has failure as an unconscious goal. Maybe she was told she was stupid or that she wouldn't amount to much as a child. That idea became fixed in her mind as a core belief and now feeds back into her daily behaviour so that she unconsciously sabotages her own success.

With the help of hypnosis, you can choose whether to be in control of where you direct your energy or whether to let it go on automatic pilot. You can direct it towards success (whatever success is for you) or anything else you may desire, and it will help you achieve it; or you can let it direct itself towards destructive goals. Since the energy itself is neither positive nor negative, it is up to you to direct it to work for or against you.

Hypnosis is the most effective way to harness the power of the subconscious in a controlled way. Of course, there are other ways of accessing it; a similar state of mind is induced when people are sick, endangered, or frightened, or because of long-distance running, dancing, repetitive chanting, spinning, and when remembering events or reviewing dreams.

Even though we can access the same state of mind in other ways, hypnotherapy works because it harnesses the power of the subconscious in a direct, guided, and controlled way.

In this chapter, I have delved into the differences between the conscious, subconscious, and unconscious mind, explored the many functions of the subconscious, and explained why hypnosis is the best way to access it. In the next chapter, I shall discuss how to induce hypnosis and provide a done-for-you script to use in the sessions that follow in part II.

Chapter 6

How to Induce Hypnosis

How to use self-hypnosis effectively

Now, let's take a brief look at how to effectively hypnotise yourself.

A typical session consists of four stages, namely:

1. Induction

2. Deepening

3. Various techniques to achieve pre-decided goals

4. Awakening

Hypnosis is created during the induction when the subject is induced into a light hypnotic state followed by the deepening which is the time when a deeper state of hypnosis is reached.

After the deepening phase comes the interesting part. This is when various techniques are used to achieve your pre-determined goals. In this case, the goal is to overcome performance anxiety. One might assume that suggestions are all that is used in this part of the session, but this would be a gross oversimplification.

Skilled hypnotherapists use a plethora of interactive techniques to create change in clients. Hypnotherapy is an art, because each client is different and a good therapist will use specific techniques customised to each client and the requirements of the session, even if the general procedure might be very similar for similar ailments. This is to ensure the therapy is well timed and fits the client's personality and needs. However, in this course I have included all the different techniques I know to help someone with this specific issue so that you can rest assured you shall be successful no matter what.

After the 'meat and potatoes' part of the session is over, you will be guided back to normal conscious awareness and helped to transition smoothly to everyday external reality. This structure is always used in any type of hypnosis although the length of each phase may differ.

If you want to hypnotise yourself you need to follow the above structure. I shall include an example of a full induction and deepening as well as the standard awakening procedure below. However, feel free to use your own if you prefer. You can find lots of books on this subject as well as free scripts on the internet. [6]

Another method of self-hypnosis is to guide yourself without a formal induction. If you have been to a self-hypnosis class, you will know how to do this. If you choose to use this method, I would recommend recording a 5 to 10-minute gap at the beginning of your recordings before you begin your suggestions.

How to induce hypnosis

Before you start, please be aware that if you are using self-hypnosis recordings at night—unless you are quite anxious and find it hard to relax—it is better not to listen to them in bed, or you may fall asleep. Instead, sit on a comfortable chair with your back and neck straight. If the tendency is to let your head drop down, don't let it; you don't want to be drowsy and you may give yourself a stiff neck otherwise. Don't slouch either. Instead, try to get the support you need.

---

[6] You can find some free scripts in the link below. However, I would advise you stay with the inductions and deepeners and not use the suggestive scripts as some of them are not top quality. https://www.hypnotistentertainment.com/wp-content/uploads/2012/07/Rene-Bastarache-American-School-of-Hypnosis-Hypnosis-Scripts-I-2008.pdf

You can use meditation cushions if you are a meditator and it feels familiar and comfortable to you. If you are sitting on a chair or lying down, make sure you keep your feet flat on the floor and your legs and arms uncrossed. Always use the same position so your body will learn to associate the posture with self-hypnosis.

Whether you are listening to your recording at night, early in the morning, or during a break in the day, make sure you switch off your mobile notifications, close social media, and avoid all distractions by putting your phone on airplane mode. You could put a sign on the door so you are not interrupted and if there are sounds around you, tell yourself you are going to ignore them, as if they came from a TV playing in another room with the volume turned down. Imagine they are a background soundtrack to your relaxation, helping you zone in on your inner world.

Step 1: Adopt the hypnotic mindset

As already mentioned in the previous chapter, to access hypnosis, you need to adopt the 'hypnotic mindset'. Let us now explore this concept further:

Expect success

Believe that hypnosis is going to happen. Expect it to work, and don't test it or hope it will work. Expressing hope implies you are doubting the effectiveness of the procedure.

Have a positive attitude

Trust yourself to be receptive. Tell yourself you are responding to the suggestions you are hearing. Be gently encouraging with yourself. Believe you can produce results without trying very hard at all.

In fact, don't *try*. *Trying* implies failure. Remember to focus. Keep it positive or it won't work! Remind yourself you are creating hypnosis by engaging your imagination. It is your choice to do so. You are doing this because you believe hypnosis serves your best interests and you are going to benefit from the session. Realise that you are in control of the process. Tell yourself you are capable and commit time and effort to the process. Be patient.

Watch your language

Keep your language simple, direct, and positive. Use emphatic words. Imagine you are talking to a bright eight-year-old. Go slow. Take your time. Speak to yourself as if you were trying to soothe a child. You wouldn't shout or speak rapidly, would you?

Pretend it is working until it does

Behave as if you already are hypnotised. Act like it. Convince yourself. Adopt the posture and the position of someone who is hypnotised. Tell yourself you are and your body will believe you and respond accordingly.

When you are ready to record the induction, remember to use a gentle and assured tone. Be encouraging and take it slow. Resist the urge to rush; instead, feel each word, and as you speak into your recording device, imagine how long it would take for you to respond to your suggestions. Be absorbed in the process. When you listen to the recording, trust you are doing this the way that is right for you. Being as still as possible will enable you to be more focused on the hypnotic process.

Step 2: Breathing exercise

Once you have assumed your chosen position, take a deep breath through your nose. Count to 4 on the inhale, hold the breath for the count of 4, exhale out for the count of 4, and again hold the breath for 4.

Each time you inhale, imagine calm entering your body and spreading through every muscle and nerve. As you exhale, imagine letting go of any stress or tension. If you like, imagine a colour you associate with calmness spreading through your body every time you breathe in. As you breathe out, imagine letting go of any tension like water flowing down the drain, and being released out of your body through your feet and fingertips. Use your imagination to change this any way it works for you. Repeat six times or as long as you need to feel the calming effect of this kind of breathing.

Step 3: The induction

The following can be used as a script. Record it word for word or add your own flavour to it.

Eye fixation

Without moving from your position, imagine looking at a real or imagined spot located as high as possible in front of you. Keeping your head still, allow your eyeballs to roll up as if you were looking in between your eyebrows. Do not bend your neck or tilt the head; keep it straight. As you fix your eyes in this way, concentrate your attention only on the spot and you will feel your eyes quickly becoming tired.

If your eyelids start fluttering, it's a good sign. Breathe in while keeping your eyes on the spot with your eyeballs rolled up. Breathe out. As you take another breath in imagine that your eyelids are getting heavier. Tell yourself they want to close and imagine how wonderfully comfortable it will be when they do. Breathe out. Keep your gaze fixed without moving at all and again take a third breath in while keeping your eyeballs up. Imagine you are so tired you are trying to fight sleep but your body wants to drift off.

You are now feeling increasingly relaxed with each breath you take. Remember what it's like to feel so drowsy and sleepy; your eyelids feel heavy and want to close. As soon as your eyes are ready to close let them and as they do, keep your eyeballs up and notice the fluttering sensation in your eyes. Now, drop your chin just a fraction so you get that looking down feeling you would experience if you were looking down a flight of stairs. Then allow your eyeballs to go back to your normal position.

The magnets

You can now show yourself the power of your wonderful imagination. Rub the palms of your hands together really fast until you notice the heat and 'energy' in between them. Hold your hands in front of you with the palms facing each other. Allow them to be about fifteen centimetres apart.

When you are ready, imagine that there are two very powerful magnets placed on each palm, drawing the hands together in an irresistible way. The idea is to allow the magnetic force in between your palms to work its magic as you imagine the force acting on both palms, irresistibly drawing them together.

Remember that you are not moving the palms together in a voluntary way, but you are also not resisting that movement. You are only letting your imagination do that for you by allowing the muscles to respond automatically. Fully engage your imagination and see, feel, and sense that magnetic force pulling your hands together.

Pretend you can feel it happening while saying to yourself internally, "With every breath I take, my hands are irresistibly drawing together, pulled in by the force of the magnets. I can try to stop it, but the harder I try, the more the hands are pulled together. As soon as your hands touch, let them drop into your lap like a dead weight.

The staircase deepener

Now that your hands are in your lap, imagine you are at the top of a beautiful staircase. See what your eyes would see, and hear what your ears would hear, and feel what you would feel as you fully imagine this scene. See and sense the staircase. What does it look like?

Now, as I count down from 10 down to 1, with each number you count, take one step down the staircase, and become sleepier and more comfortable with each step. Take step 10, and as you do feel your feet, see your feet, hear your feet treading each step down.

Every step takes you deeper into hypnosis. The deeper you go, the better you feel, and the better you feel, the deeper you go. Now, take step 9 and as you do, allow yourself to feel how heavy and comfortable you are becoming. Give yourself permission to let go. It is safe to unwind, because you are in complete control.

Now, take step 8 and go deeper. And deeper means going deeper into a deeper awareness of your inner self. So, go deeper, drift deeper, sleep deeper. And sleep just means sleep of the nervous system so you can allow yourself to feel more naturally calm and peaceful than you've ever felt before.

Now, take step 7. And as you tune into your body, feel which parts of your body are feeling the most comfortable and calm. It may be a part that's feeling particularly heavy, or particularly light, or maybe a part that doesn't feel much at all. Like the deeper part of a pond, still in the moonlight, let your mind be focused on my voice, the sound of my voice and the pauses in between the words.

And now, take step 6, and tell yourself every sound, inside or outside the room, any movement, only serves to enhance your experience of relaxation, like a background soundtrack to your comfort, or a TV with the sound turned all the way down. And if any thoughts drift in and out of your consciousness, let them be what they are, and then focus back on my words. It's all part of the process.

Now, take step 5, half way down. Tell yourself you are responding so well, you are so focused, you choose to trust you are doing this in the right way for you today. You are protected, you are safe, you are going deeper and deeper into a wonderful hypnotic sleep. You are so engrossed in the process; you notice all the details of shade and light and you are floating down that staircase like water on oil.

Now, take step 4. Sleep deeper. Go deeper. Drift deeper. Allow yourself to soften your body. Perhaps you see a relaxing colour spread through your body, one muscle at a time. Now, take step 3. And as you do, imagine that colour relaxing you deeply, but only as much as you want to. Imagine what those muscles would look and feel like from the inside if they were loose and limp and relaxed.

Now, take step 2 and it's like you are watching a movie of yourself becoming so engrossed, so at ease, like when you are watching a movie or reading your favourite book and you are so connected with the characters and the story, you are so absolutely absorbed in the experience of being in this wonderful feeling of calm and peace. It's like nothing else in the world matters right now...

And now, take step 1. As you do, it's like you can see yourself from above, watching yourself in this moment. You are so aware of yourself that you can imagine what you look like in the position you are in. It's like you could float up and you could look down at your body there.

And as you leave the building where your body is in, as you float up and explore and you are going higher and higher, you are going deeper and deeper into hypnosis and you see life going on down there, observing the landscape as you travel higher.

Now you start to see the larger land mass and even the coastline, and you see less and less details of the streets below as you float higher and higher through the clouds and beyond the atmosphere until you see the entire planet earth in front of you. You can see the planet in its amazing beauty from here in outer space.

And as you notice the different perspective you have here, you can see the earth and all life within it, and you begin to understand more about yourself and life. You begin to benefit from the wisdom of the universe. You begin to gain insight and perspective from this higher place.

Suggestions and change work

Here, add your own autosuggestions or use the techniques and strategies that are outlined in each of the sessions in part II, III, and IV (Audio sessions 1-10).

61

Exit from hypnosis

Now it's time to come out of hypnosis. As you count from 1 to 5, imagine going up a flight of stairs and with each and every number you count, you become more awake, more aware, and at the count of 5, you are fully awake and aware and back to your normal conscious awareness.

Number 1, easily and gently begin returning to your full conscious awareness. Number 2, more and more awake and aware with each number that I count. Number 3, normal sensations are coming back now, feeling good in mind and body, bringing all the benefits of this session to your everyday life. Number 4, wiggling your toes and your fingers, getting ready to open your eyes. Number 5, eyes open, feeling good mentally, physically, and emotionally.

Once your eyes are open, take your time before you drive a car or operate any machinery. Take it easy, allowing for the transition between hypnosis and normal life to happen at your own pace.

In this chapter, I have shown you the practical steps for you to take in order to successfully hypnotise yourself. In the next chapter, I will show you how other people with performance anxiety have benefited from my hypnotic sessions so you can see how change is not only possible but inevitable when you know how to bring it about.

Chapter 7

Case Studies

In this section, I shall illustrate how hypnotherapy has served some of my performance anxiety clients extremely well by lifting them up from insecurity and worry to confidence and stage presence. Some of them felt nervous performing music in public, and others had difficulties with public speaking, interviews, auditions, and exams. Some had a fear of not being able to learn lines, and some felt very anxious about practicing in front of others and learning new material. Regardless of their situation, hypnotherapy helped them regain their power to move forward in life.

Please note that all names and any other identifiable details have been changed to protect the clients' identities.

Lisa James: a world class drummer afraid to go on tour

Lisa James was in her early forties when she came to see me. She was a highly accomplished drummer who taught music for a living and had been playing with a successful band in her twenties, but had taken a break since. She came to see me because her old band was going on a world tour and wanted her to return as their drummer. This was a lifelong dream for Lisa and she wanted nothing more than to be reunited with her best friends to play music in front of thousands of people.

However, the prospect of playing in front of big crowds terrified her. Now, the stakes were so high that she felt scared of messing up, making mistakes, and forgetting what she was doing. That would be a disaster! After taking her case history, it became apparent that Lisa was very fond of 'what ifs' and struggled with catastrophic thinking, anxiety, and depression, especially since she had lost her father at the age of seventeen.

In her initial interview, Lisa mentioned that her mother had always been very hard on her, taking everything extremely seriously and wouldn't speak to her for days if she failed at sports. She remembered feeling anxious when playing volleyball and her mother was around to watch her. She was now due to either accept or reject the offer of her old band and she felt very low, confused, anxious, hopeless, and sometimes even suicidal.

It was immediately clear to me that although Lisa was highly skilled as a drummer and capable of touring with her band, the problem lay primarily with the fear of making mistakes; so I decided that we needed to understand where she had learned that it was not okay to make mistakes. We focussed on the feeling of fear around this and after hypnotising her, I asked her to return to the very first time she could remember feeling that way. She easily recalled an incident during a volleyball training session where her mother had been particularly critical of her performance and had ridiculed her in front of her peers for 'messing up'.

It was now clear that this traumatic experience was responsible for the unconscious learning she had incorporated into her belief system about the dangers of making mistakes. If ridicule and withdrawal of love follows messing up, then this will be encoded as a threat to the individual. In these circumstances, it is important to reframe traumatic past events in a way that can be helpful and empowering.

I asked adult Lisa to go back to the incident and comfort little Lisa in the way she would have wanted to be comforted. I also asked her to explore any unresolved feelings towards her mother. I then asked her to rewrite the story from an empowered perspective so she could learn how to parent herself in a more helpful, compassionate, and gently encouraging way. This kind of work helped her reframe the misconception that it is not ok to make mistakes, and to see her mother's critical attitude as a misguided attempt to make her a good sportswoman. The process described above is a mixture of Inner Child Therapy and Regression and it is partly reproduced in Bonus Session 2: Letting go of fear of rejection.

Now that the primary cause of anxiety had been identified and dealt with, we focussed on replacing negative habits of worrying and catastrophising before performances with the positive habit of staying in the present. We worked on installing a present focussed mindset, insisting that the only thing that matters is the current moment because the past is gone and the future is yet to be created by positively and meaningfully living in the 'now'.

We built confidence by encouraging her to pay particular attention to her creative expression and enjoyment of the piece. We reprogrammed her mind by resetting it to the default program of simply enjoying playing music, which was how she felt before her mother had ever criticised her. I also asked Lisa to think of a drummer who had the qualities she admired and who was very relaxed and confident on stage. Since we learn by modelling others, it is important to identify someone to aspire to so we can channel those qualities in ourselves. The techniques described above are contained in part III of this book.

On our third session, I taught Lisa self-hypnosis and asked her to practice diaphragmatic breathing every day so she could learn how to calm herself down whenever she experienced symptoms of anxiety. During hypnosis, I elicited a calm state of mind and asked her to anchor it to a physical gesture she could use any time she wanted to recapture the same state in everyday life.

To help her feel safe, I asked her to select a positive and helpful statement that would remind her to come back to the present every time she felt drawn into a fantasy of the future. I then instructed her on how to use it while imagining the positive outcome she wanted during performances instead of the one she feared.

We also worked on how to regain flow so that even if she did make a mistake or became self-conscious during a song, she could easily bring herself back to what really mattered. I asked her to practice all the techniques we learnt by listening to our recorded sessions daily. (The above techniques can be learned in Audio sessions 1, 3, 5, and 9.)

Since Lisa felt a lot better after our fourth session, we decided to focus on physical ways of embodying the new mindset she had just learned. I taught her about 'power poses'—a way in which the body can teach our mind to feel calm and empowered.

I also taught her how to shake tension out of her body before a performance, how to ground herself, how to align herself energetically and how to feed off her power centre so she could feel fully present in her body and gain stage presence. She informed me she was now ready to say yes to the opportunity of a lifetime, and was feeling elated and excited.

A few months later I spoke with Lisa and asked her how the tour had gone. She said:

"I'm doing great! I played many concerts since I saw you and although I still get a little niggle at times, I'm fine, I find the biggest difference is that I don't worry about shows before they happen anymore. I've even done live TV in front of a studio audience... that would have really freaked me out in the past. Even better, after only two weeks out our album went to number 1 in the album charts!"

Tim Fraser: "everyone is against me!"

Tim was a shy, introspective, and introverted environmental health student who came to me because he felt anxious giving presentations and wanted to do his best for his dissertation so he could get a good job once he graduated from university. I asked him what stood in his way of presenting, and the strongest obstacle seemed to be fear of judgement and failure.

He would feel very nervous before presentations, avoiding food, or throwing up, especially when comparing himself to other students and finding himself wanting. During presentations, his mind would often go blank, his face red, he would speak too fast, reading slides and imagining others would judge him to be boring.

When I asked about his lifestyle, Tim said he smoked cannabis daily to soothe anxiety and had done so since he was a teen when he had been expelled from school due to a cannabis-related incident. Although it had been tough at the time, the experience seemed to have been positive overall. At school, he hadn't worked very hard, but he had excelled in sports and he now loved his course.

Digging a little deeper, I learned Tim had lost confidence going to college as it had been a big change from boarding school and making friends had not been as easy. He also felt that his teachers were against him at times, and he would not be able to stay at a school for longer than two or three years before things would 'boil up' and he'd be expelled. Work-wise, he had tried to secure a job he really liked, but hadn't gone past the interview stage due to his nervousness.

I asked him how he had managed to cope so far, and he said he had tried shaking off tension, controlling his breathing, and standing up straight, but it hadn't been enough. It seemed that although he felt he had always been shy, he was confident about his sports ability and he believed himself to be smart. The trouble lay in second guessing himself and worrying about what other people thought about him.

I explained to Tim that when we imagine others are judging us, it is often a projection of our own self judgement. Often, this is caused by events where others have judged us harshly and we have internalised the criticism to avoid being vulnerable and going through a similar situation again. Given that Tim already seemed to be familiar with calming breathing techniques, we started our sessions focusing on mindset instead.

The best way to stop obsessing about the idea of others criticising us, is to focus on something else which is more positive and closer to reality. Therefore, during hypnosis, I asked Tim to reframe the presentation process as an opportunity to share his knowledge and expertise, focussing on the message he was passionate about and placing his mind in the present.

After this initial session, we proceeded to explore whether his previous experiences with presentations had been traumatic enough to imprint as a threat. To clear any unsavoury associations that may cause him to respond similarly in future situations, we used the LAMA method which I developed to help people let go of the past. See Part III for details of what this entails.

During the next couple of sessions, we focused on creating a better future for Tim by rehearsing what that would look like in terms of giving presentations. The idea was to only take from the past what was useful and to let go of the rest. The second step was to focus on enjoying delivering information and appreciating that the teachers' aim was to get the best for their students. This idea seemed to resonate particularly well with him. When he woke up from the 'trance' he had had a realisation: what he really needed to let go of was the idea that everyone—and especially teachers—were against him!

This new understanding left Tim feeling much more confident. He felt different now, almost as if he had found the missing piece of a jigsaw puzzle. In our last session, we explored and reframed the concept of failure, seeing it as an opportunity to learn something new. We changed the definition of success from the idea of being approved of externally by others, to internally approving of oneself for doing one's best. When viewing situations from this lens, there really is no failure until you quit or give up on yourself, and even then, there is a beneficial lesson to be learned which can help you do better in the long run.

Tim left our sessions a changed young man. He even looked different in the way he walked out the door. He seemed taller to me, as if he had grown up into the adult he had only dreamed of being before.

Andrew Smith: "what if I forget my lines?"

Andrew was a 53-year-old actor and writer who came to me because he had been chosen for a part in a play and rehearsals were due to start in two weeks. He felt very anxious about not being able to learn his lines in time and was fearful of letting the director and the other actors down. He felt his age wasn't on his side; he thought of himself as slow and spent a lot of time imagining the worst-case scenario.

Part of the problem was that although he had previously worked in film, it had been years since his last theatre job. I asked him about his motivation for overcoming his problem and he said that this job was the beginning of a new career for him. Since his kids had now grown up, he was ready to get back into acting full time. His dream was to play leading parts in good theatre shows.

The problem was that Andrew felt out of his comfort zone. Film work had been made easier by the fact that his wife was a well-known actress with many contacts. In theatre on the other hand, he had few contacts and there was no 'second take'. I asked him what his relationship with his wife was like—just to cover all angles and ensure there were no jealousies or conflicts. On the contrary, it seemed as though she was an inspiration for him. I decided to make use of this detail in our later sessions to turn his admiration to his own advantage.

There didn't seem to be any traumatic events in Andrew's past that could have contributed to his fear of forgetting lines. It also seemed that Andrew did not have a problem with memory in general. He was perfectly capable of recalling books he had read, phone numbers, directions, and shopping lists. My bet was the issue did not lie with his memory, but with an interference in recall due to anxiety.

Despite his obvious competence, what seemed to stop him was the bad habit of worrying, catastrophic thinking, and worrying about worrying. When we worry, our minds become obsessed with a specific negative thought. This process demands all our attention and if done long enough can cause negative physiological changes that interfere with memory recall.

Have you ever had the experience of someone asking you for the name of a specific person only for that name to suddenly slip out of reach? The more upset you become about the fact that you can't remember it, and the more you try to consciously remember it, the less successful you will be. Your best bet is to relax and think about something else and suddenly, there it is! This is because when we relax, we give our subconscious mind a chance to do the work for us. It is only when we interfere with it out of mistrust or fear, that we stop it from doing what it does best—giving us what we ask for.

In the light of this information, I decided that the key to Andrew's treatment was to teach him how to relax and how to use his vivid imagination in a beneficial way. In our first session, I trained him in self-hypnosis and taught him how to breathe through his diaphragm. Then I showed him how to turn his thinking around so he would start imagining what he wanted, rather than the contrary. We practiced positive mental rehearsal of the event, focusing on staying in the present, connecting with the message of his lines, and enjoying performing. (All the above techniques are described in detail in Audio Session 1, 3, and 7.)

After successfully completing these tasks, I showed Andrew an exercise called 'thought stopping'. This effectively replaces negative thoughts associated with a particularly triggering situation with heart-centred thinking and allows us to nip catastrophic imagining in the bud. Fear is transformed into trust. (You can find this technique in Audio Session 8.)

Finally, in our last session, I focussed on increasing Andrew's confidence by helping him recall and relive peak experiences in his film work when he felt competent and remembered his lines well. This redressed the balance in his mind, reminding him he already had the skills required within himself. I taught him a way to anchor these positive experiences in his body so he could use their memory to trigger the same confident state of mind at will. (You can find this process described in Audio Session 10.)

By learning to use his imagination well, calm his body, and trust in himself, Andrew was able to learn all his lines in two weeks—stress free. I went to see his show and he performed excellently.

Casey Ford: "if I let go, I may drown..."

Casey was a 25-year-old opera singer studying at music school. She came to me wanting to be able to emotionally connect with the music she was performing. She believed her upbringing was responsible for holding her back. She had left the strictly religious community in which she was raised when she'd turned eighteen. She felt she had been brainwashed and emotionally abused as well as bullied by her family. Feelings were not only not welcomed at home, but any kind of emotional expression was severely punished. Her siblings also suffered psychological trauma and had developed dysfunctional behaviours including an eating disorder, self-harm, drug abuse, and threats of violence.

Her father had an anger problem, and both he and her mother were depressed. Casey herself had previously suffered from depression. She had been made to feel inadequate all her life, not living up to the dream of perfection her family and community set out for her. She felt sinful and wished she could be killed for her faith to atone for her sins. She had realised this line of thinking to be faulty only when she had told her sister about it.

In terms of music school, she had been a bright kid, but her undergraduate studies had suffered due to her struggle with depression and she had begun to lose her voice in her final year. She felt she had been treated unfairly by the head of department, who sabotaged her scholarship for personal reasons. This event had caused her to pull out of singing engagements, lose motivation, and give up altogether on her singing career.

Despite all these difficulties, Casey had decided to get back on track. She had just hired a new singing teacher, enrolled in an acting course, was studying piano and martial arts, and felt like a phoenix rising from the ashes of destruction. Her ultimate goal was to perform in Covent Garden, La Scala, or the Bolshoi. I had a strong feeling of compassion and affection for Casey, who seemed to be a sensitive young woman who had been through a lot, but was determined not to let her experience make a victim out of her.

She had already done some hypnotherapy to deal with her emotional issues and it had worked. Now, she faced a disconnection from the music she was singing. She felt afraid of really connecting with the emotions the music elicited and letting herself feel them.

I asked her, "What would happen if you did allow yourself to connect with your feelings?"

"I am afraid I might just drown."

This suggested to me that Casey had been repressing her emotions for so long that she felt she might become overwhelmed if she allowed herself to 'go there'.

In light of this understanding, I decided to deal with her fear of 'drowning' first. Using 'Inner Child Therapy' and my own method for trauma release (see Bonus Audio Sessions 1 and 2), we cleared the unconscious pattern of avoidance Casey had adopted to keep herself safe. She was now able to reframe what had happened to her and see her fear as a response to a dysfunctional situation in which she needed to protect herself in the only way she knew how at the time. Consequently, she could create a new, updated pattern that would serve her better in the present so she would respond differently to triggers that once would have seen her stuck in her past conditioning.

In our second session, we used a process that allowed Casey to let go of the past and feel able to 'swim' in the river of her emotions (See Audio Session 4 for a description of this). Once able to give herself permission to feel pain without feeling overwhelmed, she could also allow other emotions to surface and inform her singing. Using mental rehearsal, I helped Casey to see herself behaving in the way she wanted, rather than in her 'old ways'. She felt free, relaxed, and safe while expressing the feeling of the music through the conduit of her voice. (This process is described in Audio Session 3 and 7.)

Having had great results in the first few sessions, Casey started to feel confident enough to apply for auditions at the higher levels, so we started to work on her stage presence. Here we used energetic and embodiment practices to shift her awareness from her head to her power centre—what some call the "Dantien", which is situated two inches below the navel—allowing her to feel grounded. These practices taught her how to feel the difference between shrinking and spilling energy, as well as very practical ways of connecting with the power of her feminine essence in its fullness.

Finally, in our last session, we used movement improvisation to practice presence so she could use the techniques learned for her character work. I taught her some power poses as well as simple Qigong exercises to help her stay calm during auditions. As a result, her singing teacher felt a dramatic shift in her abilities and Casey was able to leave therapy feeling very confident and determined to audition in the UK as well as Europe.

Amanda Swift: "I'll be rejected just like I was back then..."

Amanda was a 54-year-old university lecturer who called me because she had been offered a speaking gig at a very prestigious event, but she felt that—despite her many years of experience with lecturing and public speaking—she lacked belief in herself. Self-doubt plagued her almost daily and when she phoned me to enquire about my services, she felt so forlorn that she burst into tears within five minutes of talking to me.

Amanda told me she went to work every day wearing a mask. Although she looked confident, she felt like an impostor. She said the problem had started when her first husband had broken off the marriage many years prior. Subsequently, she had remarried, but when a priest had chastised her for wanting to do so, she had felt the wound reopen. Recently, her ex had been back in touch and that's when she had begun to feel overwhelmed.

It was clear to me that there was an important connection between these events and her issue, so I sought to explore the matter further. When I asked Amanda what was the worst that could happen at the gig, she said she was scared the audience would judge her and reject her just like *he did*. Here was the key to the puzzle. After a little more digging into the circumstances of their breakup, it became apparent that Amanda had felt deeply wounded by her ex-husband's betrayal and abandonment.

After many years of marriage, he had suddenly announced to her that he had fallen for someone else and had left her with three kids to raise on her own while he travelled abroad to start a new life. This event created what I call *negative learning* around her identity and core beliefs. She started thinking she had been rejected because she was worthless and 'not good enough'. This belief was then exacerbated by the priest's severe judgement when she asked his opinion about remarrying. In short, the traumatic event of her ex leaving had been encoded as a dangerous threat, and anything that matched it in form (such as situations that might cause further rejection) would be followed by anxiety and panic.

This theory was further confirmed when I asked Amanda about where she felt strong and confident and she mentioned the many positive talks she had given and the many places she had travelled alone with her kids.

Knowing this, it became apparent that what needed to happen was for Amanda to reframe what had happened with her ex, so the balance could be restored by a fairer perspective.

She needed to see that his leaving had nothing to do with her and more to do with him, and she needed to see how she was worthy of love and belonging, regardless of whether she was perfect or not. After working on the trauma, we focused on building positive self-talk centred on the idea of self-acceptance, self-compassion, and kindness. We then worked with limiting beliefs—transforming them from disempowering statements into empowering deeper truths. You will find out how to do the same in Bonus Session 3.

Once a positive mindset was established, we proceeded to reframe the speaking gig itself. The aim of the work was to break with any negative past experiences related to speaking and create a more balanced and accurate view of what a good experience of speaking in public is all about. We focussed on sharing knowledge, authentic expression, and enjoyment as well as staying in the present. (You can find an example of this type of session in Audio Session 7.)

Finally, we thoroughly rehearsed her ideal outcome until she felt confident about delivering her speech. After our sessions were over, Amanda got back in touch saying the engagement had been cancelled, but she had applied for another one and felt confident she would now be pursuing her career with renewed confidence.

In this chapter, I have shown you how other people with similar issues to yours have overcome performance anxiety and achieved the change they wanted. You can do it too with the power of hypnosis! Now it is time to jump into the practical part of this book, where you will go through a wonderful journey of transformation and discover the joy of being seen.

In the next Chapter, I shall explain how fear and anxiety are generated and what to do to overcome them.

PART II—
SESSIONS 1-3

FINDING YOUR WAY
THROUGH THE FEAR

DOWNLOAD the Dare to Be Seen BONUS PACKAGE

including a

FREE AUDIOBOOK, CHECKLIST and WORKBOOK

Templates, Training, Resources to Kickstart your Journey into Authentic Confidence under the Spotlight!

TO DOWNLOAD GO TO
https://elisadinapoli.com/bonuses

Audio Session 1

Calming the Body and Mind

In this session, we will explore why panic happens, how it is triggered, and how to turn it off so you can feel relaxed when presenting, giving a speech, playing a gig, or going for an interview.

If you are one of those people that experiences strong physical symptoms when undertaking a task under public scrutiny, chances are you are triggering your fight or flight response. In other words, you are experiencing the beginning of what could develop into a full-fledged panic attack. The good news is that panic is one of the easiest states to defuse, provided you know what to do.

Understanding panic

To understand the panic response, we need to have a basic understanding of our brain. Roughly speaking, as humans, we possess three 'intelligence systems':

The **brain stem** corresponds to the 'movement intelligence system' which controls the movement of our body in space and regulates the central nervous system. It takes care of our breathing, heart rate, sleeping, and eating functions.

The **limbic brain** corresponds to the 'emotional intelligence system'. The thalamus gathers information such as sight and sound and sends it to both the amygdala and the neocortex.

The **amygdala** is part of the limbic system and it is the alarm centre of the brain. Its job is to respond to the information sent by the thalamus, using a process called crude pattern matching, which I will discuss in depth in chapter 8. Once the information is received, the amygdala compares it to its already stored emotional memories and divides stimuli between possible threats and emotionally satisfying experiences.

Finally, we have the **neocortex**, which is the 'thinking intelligence system'. It is involved in cognition, sensory perception, spatial reasoning, and language, and it is the executive part of the brain. This is where rational, analytical thinking happens.

Why are you afraid? —The amygdala's role

When a trigger is identified as a threat, the amygdala turns the alarm on so you can get ready to fight the threat, flee the situation, or freeze, which is tantamount to pretending you are dead. In a real-life scenario, this mechanism could save your life.

So, how does the amygdala do its job? When a threat is identified, the stress hormones cortisol and adrenaline are pumped into your bloodstream. You start breathing fast and shallow in an attempt to pump more oxygen into your body so you are ready for aerobic exercise.

Blood rushes from the extremities into your heart so you can run or fight with as much energy as possible. Your heart is pounding, your heart rate is increased, and you may start to sweat profusely. This is because sweating is your body's way of trying to control temperature when aerobic exercise is expected. If you aren't faced with a *real*-life threat, but only an imagined one, you can start hyperventilating.

What is hyperventilation and why is it important to avoid it?

Hyperventilation happens when the body is preparing for aerobic exercise, such as during the fight or flight response; but since there is no real threat, we do not fight or run. In this case, we are taking in more oxygen than we need by breathing in rapid short in and out breaths. Too much breathing out causes too much carbon dioxide to leave the body. Basically, you are breathing out too much CO_2. Since CO_2 is needed by the body to metabolise oxygen so the latter can be carried to your body's tissues, not enough oxygen will reach them and you will experience some or all of the following symptoms:

Lightheadedness
Giddiness
Dizziness
Shortness of breath
Heart palpitations
Numbness
Chest pains
Dry mouth
Clammy hands
Difficulties in swallowing
Tremors
Sweating
Weakness
Fatigue

These symptoms can be scary, and not knowing why you are feeling this way can fuel the panic response, but rest assured, they are only temporary. Another common symptom of hyperventilation is nausea or abdominal distress. According to some evolutionary psychologists, this is an ancient defence mechanism designed to put off animals that might be attacking you, as vomit or excrement might suggest you are not a suitable prey.

Psychologically, you may also experience 'de-realisation' which is when you find yourself thinking, *'this is not real'*. This is a defence mechanism designed to cap anxiety, ensuring you don't experience a heart attack out of fear.

Unfortunately, the thought of having a heart attack can lead you to believe you are about to have one, especially when coupled with the feeling of not being able to breathe, experiencing chest pain, or being afraid of losing control. Although the fear of having it can fuel the panic, it is very unlikely you will have an actual heart attack.

The other common fear that feeds panic is the belief that you could suffocate or that you could faint. Suffocation is out of the question without an obstructing object and the only reason you are feeling that way, is because you are hyperventilating. Fainting would also be very unusual during a panic attack, because blood is being pumped very fast and you cannot faint unless the heart slows down.

You may also become so worked up that you feel convinced you are having a nervous breakdown, but the reality is that there is no such thing. This is an outdated metaphor used to describe psychiatric disorders and it only serves to frighten people. It is much more likely you are experiencing a stress overload because one or more of your emotional needs are under threat (such as the need for safety) and as soon as the trigger is gone, you will feel normal. This is made obvious by the fact that as soon as you remove yourself from the threatening scenario, you will start to feel better.

You may also believe you are going to be embarrassed or humiliated and that further encourages panic. What you need to remember is that nothing bad can happen as a direct result of embarrassment. What makes it a problem is the meaning you give it. If you choose to laugh at yourself a little and take yourself less seriously, you will realise an embarrassing situation can be so ridiculous as to become hilarious.

How fear makes you stupid...

While all of this may make rational sense to you, it is not possible to think clearly at the height of panic. This is because when you become highly emotionally aroused—such as when your fight or flight response is triggered—information received by your sensory system is fast tracked to the amygdala without first passing through the 'thinking brain'—the neocortex.

This is known as 'emotional hijacking' and it is a mechanism that would have served us well in the wild. Back in the day, if you suddenly met a boar, you would not sit down and reason with it or ponder whether it is going to kill you or not. The faster you reacted to the threat, the more likely you were to survive.

Likewise, when you find yourself in a situation that has been labelled as dangerous,

effectively, you will start thinking in less nuanced ways. You will make quick decisions and begin to think in black and white, life or death, and all or nothing terms. Although this would work in the wild where you need to make split second decisions, in our modern society, it means your intelligence is being inhibited, and you are unable to think rationally. So, if you are in a panic and someone tries to convince you that there is nothing to worry about, their rational arguments won't have much effect on you until you have calmed down.

This is because when you are in fight or flight mode, the alarm is effectively on, and until you turn it off, your capacity for rational thinking is at an all-time low. So, how do you turn it off? Imagine a double switch. One turns the lamp on at your desk, and the other turns the bedside light on. When you turn one on, the other switches off. The same happens in our bodies.

In panic mode, the sympathetic nervous system is on, which means the parasympathetic nervous system is off. Conversely, the latter is on when we rest or relax. Only one of the two can be on at any one time, so the best way to switch off the alarm is to turn on the parasympathetic nervous system.

How do I stop a panic attack?

So, how do you turn on the parasympathetic nervous system? The first step is to stop hyperventilating. To do so, you need to increase the levels of carbon dioxide in the blood. There are 4 ways of doing that:

1. Hold your breath a few times for 10-15 seconds intervals, to prevent the dissipation of CO_2 until symptoms subside.

2. Breathe in and out of a paper bag (covering the nose and mouth) or alternatively, breathe in and out of a straw. This will quickly restore PH levels. Note: this is not recommended for asthmatics.

3. Engage in vigorous aerobic exercise while breathing in and out of the nose. Try running up and down the stairs ten times, or doing burpees or star jumps (unless you have asthma or other diseases, in which case you should disregard this advice). Vigorous exercise will not only stop the panic attack, but it will prove to you that you are not having a heart attack. Engaging in this activity will enable you to burn more oxygen and manufacture more carbon dioxide. It will also tell your body the threat is over and that it's now time to recover.

4. Engage in deep diaphragmatic breathing for at least 5 minutes. With your shoulders down, allow your stomach to expand as you take a deep breath in through the nose, and fill up your lungs. Then exhale through the nose for twice as long as you inhaled. It is important you breathe through the nose rather than the mouth as this will reduce the amount of CO_2 entering the body.

This kind of breathing stimulates the parasympathetic nervous system and thus flicks the switch of the alarm system off. Practicing this type of breathing for 10 to 15 minutes each day, while lying down, will also help prevent panic altogether. Once the panic response is over and your body is calm, your neocortex will be back to normal and you will also be able to use positive self-talk to stay calm.

In the following session, you will learn how to switch off the fear response by calming your body and engaging the parasympathetic nervous system using the fourth method above. You will also learn how to do this at will in your everyday life using a hypnotic anchor. An anchor is a physical reminder subconsciously associated with a desired state of mind, in this case the resourceful state of calm. With this in mind, it is time to listen to your transformational hypnotic audio.

To do so, download the bonus package by typing the following link on your browser: https://tinyurl.com/daretobeseenonlinecourse

Alternatively, you can make up your own session. Begin by recording the induction and deepening as described in Chapter 6. Speak slowly and clearly into your recording device and then record the following points before finishing with the "awakening" section also described in Chapter 6.

Here is a summary of the online content:

Step 1: Relax

Find a place where you can relax and won't be disturbed. Switch off all electronic devices and either sit down with your back straight on a chair, or lie down on a bed. Keep your legs and hands uncrossed.

Engage in diaphragmatic breathing for 3 or more breaths. Every time you inhale, imagine you are inhaling relaxation and every time you exhale, imagine you are releasing tension. Relax your entire body, focussing on the feet first, and make your way up to the top of your head.

Step 2: Connect to your motivation

When you are suitably relaxed, think about why you want to overcome your anxieties around performing. Think about all the benefits you will enjoy when you achieve this. Think about how your life will change. This is your motivation and will give you fuel for the fire of change.

Step 3: Connect to your peaceful place

Imagine your mind is like a clear lake. When the water is calm, it perfectly reflects the environment that surrounds it, but if you were to throw a pebble in, it would distort reality until the water settled again. The mind is like that. When it is calm, you can make wise decisions because you see clearly. To help you calm your mind when you begin to feel disturbed, think of a peaceful place—a real or imagined place where you feel calm, safe, and at ease. Imagine it while fully engaging all your senses. When you have heightened it to the maximum degree, imagine the calm feelings you are experiencing flowing back to the thumb and a finger of your writing hand. Press them together and allow an association to be created between this gesture and the state of mind you are in right now. When the connection has been made, allow your fingers to relax.

Step 4: Positive mental rehearsal of triggering situations

Now, imagine a typical situation that would have made you feel anxious in the past. Perhaps you are waiting to go on stage, or maybe it's days before the event and you are preparing your speech or song. See yourself there and notice what kind of symptoms and feelings you have when you begin to feel anxious. As soon as you notice these feelings, use your peaceful place anchor to calm yourself. With your thumb and peaceful place finger pressed, now see yourself reacting in the way you want to react. See yourself calm, breathing deeply, and talking to yourself in a reassuring and gently encouraging way.

Step 5: Repetition

Repeat Step 4, three to five times or until you feel calmer around this particular scenario.

Step 6: Exit hypnosis

Wake yourself up by counting from 1-5. Repeat this session every day for a week or as long as you need to begin to feel the benefits. When you feel comfortable with this scenario, you can focus the session on a different one. Use this technique for any situation that arouses fear or anxiety.

Homework Session 1

After you've listened to the audio session for a few days, you can begin maximising your progress by putting into practice what you have learnt and reinforcing subconscious learning with conscious choice. Try the following:

Practice diaphragmatic breathing for a minimum of 1 to 5 minutes a day, lying down with your legs and arms uncrossed. Always breathe through your nose.

When you feel the anxiety creep in, stop whatever you are doing, tap the side of your hand lightly repeatedly and say: "Even though I am... (nervous, anxious, or scared) I deeply and completely accept and love myself anyway." Do this by tapping on the 'karate chop point'[7] of the hand.

---

[7] For a diagram illustrating the placement of this point visit
https://www.hypnotichealing.co.uk/EFT

In the next session, we will look at how accepting fear will allow you to move past it and at how to flip dominant negative worries around performing into positive power statements.

Audio Session 2

Connecting to Heart Wisdom—
the Flipping Process

Head or heart: that is the question

I believe there are two main forces inside of us that guide our decisions and shape the direction of our lives. There are many names for these two forces, depending on your belief system, so I will try to include them all here:

- the head and the heart

- the ego and the soul

- the personality and the essence

- the rational mind and the emotional self

- and if you are spiritually inclined, you and 'Spirit' or you and God, or you and your 'Higher Self'.

For ease of understanding, I shall address these concepts as Head vs. Heart, but feel free to translate that into your own words.

Your head, or your conscious, analytical, reasoning mind wants to keep you safe inside your comfort zone. Its main job is to keep you alive and away from risk. This is good to a degree, but if you only listen to your head, you will stay small and not be able to connect to what makes you feel truly alive. If you pay too much attention to your head, you will drown in fear and not be able to connect to your desire, your wisdom, or your deeper truth.

Your heart, on the other hand, wants you to expand and grow. It is not interested in comfort. When you connect to its voice, you will feel a sense of freedom and excitement, but also fear. Why? Because when you are in touch with your heart's desire, you will most definitely be out of your comfort zone and that's when your fear kicks back in and demands attention.

When you are anxious, you are mostly in your head. You are most likely in a situation that is out of your comfort zone and you are seeing it as a threat to your safety. You are judging what is happening and you are making up a story about it that scares you. You are focusing on what you could be losing and all the imaginary catastrophes that could befall you if you pursue that course of action. So, if you want to feel less anxious, you need to connect and pay attention to your heart and listen to what it has to say.

The comic and transformational speaker, Kyle Cease[8], talks about 'fearnoculars'. These are basically binoculars that limit your vision to only what you fear. When you wear them, you can only see a very limited picture of what exists and that is the picture your mind accepts as reality.

Your analytical mind is more aware of the risks of what you might be losing, rather than of possibilities of what you could be gaining. But as you step into your heart and accept all of you—including the fear, the full story with all its painful experiences—you will find that the heart is louder and wiser than the thoughts, and the more you do that, the more fear will leave you. When you are within your highest truth, you are no longer scared to leap, because it feels right.

The funny thing is when you ask your heart what the deeper truth is, the mind will come up with reasons why that truth won't work. That is a sign you are on the right path, because whenever you expand, your fear will try to make you shrink back to safety with all kinds of statements such as 'you should do this instead' or 'you shouldn't do that' or 'what if this and that goes wrong'. Your head will always find the problem in the

---

[8] Kyle Cease is the author of "The Limitation Game" https://kylecease.com/interactive/

opportunity. If you listen to it, the opportunity will go away, you will stay in the familiar, and you'll keep navigating through your personal hell.

If, instead, you resist the impulse to shrink and courageously listen to your heart, your comfort zone will expand and the fear will gradually recede. When you choose to find the opportunity in the problem, the reasons why you think you can't do what you want to do will become the reasons to do it. So, let's throw away our 'fearnoculars' and step into our heart.

Anxiety is not the problem

It is perfectly 'normal' to feel nervous when you are watched by an audience, no matter what the performance actually is. Whenever you are visible and 'centre stage', you are vulnerable. And the greatest threat for human beings has always been—and remains—peer group expulsion.

In the past, this would have been tantamount to a death sentence, because without proper support, human beings cannot survive alone—at least not for long. I would suggest this is why conformist behaviour is so common in human society. It is a normal instinct to avoid sticking our head above the parapet, in case we are kicked out of the group.

On the other hand, if we don't allow ourselves to be seen and heard, we are effectively hiding our true self and putting up an inauthentic front. Not only can this be very detrimental to our relationships and our sense of self as part of the wider community, but it can also hurt our career ambitions. Increasingly, the competitive workplace requires us to step up to leadership positions. Even getting a job requires us to stand out and be seen.

This is even more true for artists, musicians, actors, and even writers! Sometimes, this fear can get the better of us, stopping us from getting the job we want, making our work stand out or achieving our full potential. To thrive in our modern world, we need to learn to rein the fear in and lower our anxiety to an acceptable level; this is an acquired skill.

Stop fighting the fear

So, should you tell yourself not to be scared? Should you get angry at yourself when you are afraid? Should you put yourself down for giving in to fear? Although this kind of reaction is very common when we discover fear is holding us back, dealing with it this way won't work: our urge to fight fear is based on fear—we're afraid that if we don't fight it, it will never go away—and this only makes it stronger.

Instead, imagine your fear is like water in a river that wants to flow down to the sea. You may try to stop it by building a dam. This could work for a while, but if you don't allow the water through eventually, it will reach a point where the dam will either overflow or break completely. When that happens, the water will have so much force that it may destroy a lot in its wake. Feelings need to be expressed; like water, they need to flow.

Why avoidance makes fear stronger

Many of us deal with frightening situations by trying to avoid them. When we do that however, we are teaching the brain to encode those scenarios as threats. The reverse is true as well: we can train the brain to think of an actual dangerous situation as safe by repeated exposure.

Have you ever wondered why people who defuse bombs seem so calm? How can they do their job when a bomb is life threateningly dangerous? Why don't their hands tremble? These people defuse bombs on such a regular basis that their brains have encoded the experience as safe. On the other hand, the fastest way to develop a phobia is by avoidance, since the implication is that if you avoid something it is because it is dangerous, and the brain will treat it as such.

So, stop avoiding what you fear. Instead, start small. Pick something you are slightly nervous about and challenge yourself to do it while at the same time engaging in positive self-talk. Remind yourself that you can do this and you choose to feel good about it. Effectively, you are training your brain to feel more comfortable in facing challenges.

Afterwards, reward yourself. This will make you associate challenges with pleasure, and fear will turn into excitement!

Self-medication breeds addiction

When avoidance is not possible, another option we often go for is control through self-medication. When fear assails us, we want to get rid of it as quickly as possible. So, we may take beta blockers, anti-anxiety tablets, have a drink, or smoke cannabis. If a substance or behaviour seems to produce enough self-soothing, we will engage in it again. What could possibly be wrong with that? After all, if you have a toothache, you take paracetamol, right? So, why would this not work for psychological pain?

The problem with this approach is that it only works in the short term and overall, it produces addictive behaviour without resolving the problem. If you have ever tried to get rid of a toothache with paracetamol, you probably found that you needed more and more to numb the pain. Painkillers only momentarily alleviate the symptoms while the cause goes untreated; the symptoms only become worse and eventually, the drugs no longer work.

The only solution is to face the actual cause of the problem; go to the dentist and endure short term discomfort in exchange for a worthwhile result: your tooth gets a chance to heal so you can be pain free. In summary, trying to control fear or trying to avoid it are just the two sides of resistance. And resistance produces more of what you are resisting.

What you resist, persists

When you resist, you become stuck. When you don't accept where you are right now, you cannot move forward. Without acceptance, there can be no progress.

When you use verbs such as 'should' or 'ought to', you are judging yourself for simply being where you are at now and assigning blame to yourself. The guilt and the shame you feel as a result, make the situation even more challenging. It's double trouble.

Instead of resisting fear, try to accept that this is where you are at *right now*. This is different from admitting defeat and giving up on yourself; to the contrary, you can now put the energy you previously wasted on feeling bad about yourself to good use. You could start noticing how you have coped in the past. After all, if you hadn't been able to cope at all, you wouldn't be here now.

Start focussing on your strengths instead of your weaknesses. There is always a way you could have behaved that would have made things a lot worse. The fact is that you chose differently. Perhaps your choices haven't always been perfect, but you can learn to make better choices. What you focus on expands, remember? So, as you learn to appreciate your capacity to cope, you can build on those coping skills and expand them further. They are proof that you can overcome challenges.

Accept your fear

Accepting your fear is the first step to moving forward. But what does accepting fear entail? Does it mean you should just give into it? Let it control you? Freak out? Of course not! When you 'buy into fear' you are likely to get the worst of its consequences. You will fill your head with fantasies of all the things that could go wrong, believing it's all a disaster, and you are bound for humiliation, rejection, and failure.

Alternatively, you may try to control circumstances or the environment to stay safe. You may exhaust yourself by over-preparing to ensure perfection and to minimise the risk of failure. Although this approach may seem reasonable at first, it can kill your joy of performing through stress.

The reality is that we cannot control anything except our own reaction to events. We can control our attitude. We can shift our perspective, and we can choose to let go of attachment to the outcome. We can set an intention to put our best effort in and accept the rest. On the other hand, the more we try to control the uncontrollable, the more we will feel out of control, which will increase anxiety.

Accepting fear does not mean 'giving into it'. It simply means *allowing it to be without judgement*. Can you say, 'I am afraid, and it's okay'? Try it now. I mean it!

Chances are, if you have done the exercise instead of just reading it, you now feel a little lighter. The process of transformation starts with surrender. Surrender to what is not under your control and align to what is.

When you can sit with your fear like an observer and you allow yourself to explore how you are feeling, you are letting in movement and change. You are letting the river flow. You are surrendering to your reality in the moment and in doing so, you are creating space for the feeling to pass. You are using the energy that would have been wasted on resistance to create a new possibility of change.

Preparatory practical exercises

In preparation for the upcoming hypnotic session, make sure you do the following exercises one after the other. Do not skip these as they are essential to the success of the audio session.

1) Acceptance exercise

Divide a piece of paper into two columns. Now, think of a situation that makes you feel 'on the spot'—it could be an interview, an audition, giving a presentation or a speech, or performing in front of a crowd. Connect to your fear. On the left-hand column, write down what you fear:

I am scared that….
I can't do that because…

When you are done, go back to the list, and on the right-hand column, add to the corresponding sentence: *And that's okay.*

For example:

I am scared that… / I can't do…, because…

I will botch up the presentation because I'll be nervous	*And that's okay*
I cannot stop my throat from drying up	*And that's okay*
I cannot sing in public because they'll laugh at me	*And that's okay*
I will never get the job I want because I am not good enough	*And that's okay*

2) Heart connection

Divide a different piece of paper in two columns again. In the top of the left-hand column, write down:

I am worried that….
I am scared that….

For example:

I will blank out and forget my speech	
My fingers will tremble during the audition due to anxiety	
I will embarrass myself because I may faint	
They will think I am incompetent because I will make mistakes	

Fill the paper with all your worries and fears regarding the situation you have chosen to work on. You will come back to this exercise after listening to the hypnotic recording.

In the following hypnotic audio session, you will learn how to use the wisdom of your 'Heart' or 'Higher Self' to flip negative, fearful beliefs into empowering, helpful ones. I call this 'The Flipping Process'. Now, it is time to listen to the hypnotic recording.

To do so, download the bonus package by typing the following link on your browser: https://tinyurl.com/daretobeseenonlinecourse

Alternatively, you can make up your own session. Begin by recording the induction and deepening as described in Chapter 6. Speak slowly and clearly into your recording device, and then record the following points before finishing with the "awakening" section also described in Chapter 6.

Here is a summary of the online content:

Step 1: Self-hypnosis

Relax in your chosen way and hypnotise yourself.

Step 2: Connect to a positive emotion

Choose a positive emotion, such as gratitude, compassion, appreciation, love, optimism, joy, or hope. You could either remember a time when you felt that way, or you could imagine what it would be like to feel that way and visualise being enfolded in that emotion fully.

Step 3: Heart connection

Connect to the area of your heart. Put a hand on your heart if that helps.

Now, tell your heart about the first fear on the list you wrote in Exercise 2. Ask your heart what it thinks about that. What is the deeper truth you need to remember about this? What do you need to hear that will help you move forward? Listen quietly. Take your time.

If doubts swarm in, you need to relax more. Allow the answer to be informed by your positive emotion. Take more time to feel calm, and then ask again. Now, tell your heart again about your fear—your problem—around this situation. Ask it for its wisdom to flip this fear into its correspondent deeper truth.

This is the quiet voice inside of you that knows what you need to do. It is the voice that we often ignore or dismiss. It is the part of us that gets us out of trouble when we hit rock bottom. The one that tells us right from wrong when our emotions are in turmoil. This is the wise inner voice that reassures us, encourages us, and spurs us on. You may be used to doubting it. So, take your time and be patient. Listen. Believe it.

You may receive a sentence or an image. If you see an image, how would you translate it into words? If the message is a sentence, make sure it is worded in a simple, short, positive, and progressive way. This is your power statement. Make sure it is positive and expressed in the present tense. When you have the answer, make a note of it in your mind by repeating it inwardly several times, as you will use it later.

Step 4: Build a positive story around your new flip to create a new reality

Now, allow this deeper truth to inform the situation. Imagine you really took it on board. How would that make you feel? Allow this feeling to grow inside of you now. Really revel in it. Build a mental picture of your flip statement as if it's already your reality. Imagine expressing this deeper truth and connect fully with that experience. How do you feel when you accept this statement more completely? Allow yourself to connect to this feeling as if it's your reality now. Connect to the real-life scenario you feared around performance and imagine expressing this feeling within it. How would that change the way you see yourself in that scenario? Imagine advancing towards what you had previously avoided or been nervous about with confidence and calm.

Step 5: Bring yourself back to your normal awareness, and write.

Now, wake yourself up by counting from 1 to 5. Return to the heart connection exercise and follow the instructions below.

Homework Session 2

Go back to the piece of paper from Exercise 2 and fill the right-hand column as follows:

A part of me is worried that...   *But deep down my heart knows...*

For example:

I will blank out and forget my speech	*I don't have to be perfect. I can take a deep breath, take my time, and reconnect to the message*
My fingers will tremble during the audition due to anxiety	*All I need to do is focus on the feeling of the piece. When I fall in love with it, I'll make them feel in love with it too!*
I will embarrass myself because I may faint	*Even if I faint it's not the end of the world. I can cope.*
They will think I am incompetent because I will make mistakes	*I can lighten up and laugh at my own mistakes. When I make mistakes, I give others permission to be human.*

Read the sentences aloud to yourself. For example:
"A part of me is scared that I will blank out and forget my speech, but deep down, my heart knows I don't have to be perfect. I can take a deep breath, take my time, and reconnect to the message"
Notice how this makes you feel. Now, transfer your deeper truths and power statements to a piece of paper and carry it with you. Alternatively, you could set a reminder on your phone or create a screensaver on your computer. Be creative with this! Whenever your negative feelings try to return, use your peaceful place anchor, breathe deeply, and remind yourself of your

deeper truth 3 to 5 times—aloud if you can—really focussing on the meaning of the words and connecting to the positive feelings they elicit.

Listen to the transformational hypnotic audio every day and work on each sentence until you have the 'deeper truth' for each one.

In the next session, you will learn how to rehearse coping and mastery strategies as they apply to performing so that you don't just cope with performance anxiety, but master it.

Audio Session 3

Coping with Excessive Anxiety

In this session, you will learn how to cope with and eventually master anxiety in the performing arena. The approach presented here is derived from evidence-based cognitive behaviour techniques centred on positive exposure therapy.

Creating new associations: mental rehearsal explained

If you are very introverted or shy, have already worked on trauma, or spend a lot of time worrying about what you don't want to happen during a performance, then this session is for you. So, if you want to let go of any negative associations around performing, you need to create new positive expectations around the situations that trigger your anxiety. This is necessary so that old triggers can be matched to new positive responses and you can feel relaxed under those circumstances. In other words, you have to change the story you tell yourself.

For this to happen, you will need to strengthen and rehearse success patterns in which you trust your intuitive responses and learn to enjoy the process of performing instead of analysing the audience's reaction.

This can be done by mentally rehearsing the situations which make you feel nervous, and imagining yourself thinking, feeling, and behaving in a way that suits you. By rehearsing this behaviour in the 'virtual TV' of your mind, you are effectively creating new neural pathways and training yourself to feel, think, and behave in the way you are imagining.

Preparatory practical exercise

1) Create a list of scary situations

On a sheet of paper, write down situations that make you feel nervous.
For example:

- *Being asked to make a speech on the spot*
- *Arranging a booking for a gig*
- *Playing a piece in front of an audition panel*
- *Pitching a project at a meeting*

2) Grade them

After brainstorming all the situations in which you imagine feeling scared or nervous, grade them on a scale from 1 to 10. One would be a situation that makes you only slightly nervous. Ten would be the most terrifying situation you could face.

3) Put them in order

After grading all of them, put them in order from the least scary to the most frightening.
We will start addressing the situation with the lowest score.

4) Score yourself

When you think of this situation right now, how confident do you feel about coping with it on a scale of 0 to 10? Note down this number.
Now it is time to listen to your transformational hypnotic audio recording.
To do so, download the bonus package by typing the following link on your browser: https://tinyurl.com/daretobeseenonlinecourse

Alternatively, if you are already familiar with self-hypnosis and you'd rather make up your own session, begin by recording the induction and deepening as described in Chapter 6. Speak slowly and clearly into your recording device and then record the following points before finishing with the "awakening" section also described in Chapter 6.

Here is a summary of the online content:

Step 1: Relax

Take yourself into hypnosis by breathing deeply and imagining you are sitting in a comfortable chair in an elevator that is going down ten floors.

Step 2: Connect to your motivation

When you are in a deep state of relaxation and inner focus, remind yourself of the positive reasons why you are engaging in this process and what you intend to gain from it. Take a little time to acknowledge the progress you have already made from the previous session, and give yourself credit. The process of inner change has already started, so celebrate your success, however small or big it may be. Express trust in your subconscious mind doing the work for you while you don't concern yourself with the 'how'.

Step 3: Recall the triggering situation

Imagine the situation you have marked lowest, on a scale of 0 to 10, on your list. Make it real in your mind. Imagine you are there now;

see the colours, the environment, the time of day, the people around you. Fill in as many details as possible.

As you do this, notice the thoughts and feelings that you are beginning to experience. Become aware of any symptoms of distress or anxiety that emerge. Notice what they are. Is your heart beating faster? Are your palms sweating? Do you have a churning feeling in your stomach? Whatever physical symptoms you feel, really notice them.

Now, become aware of your habitual negative self-talk. Notice any critical, self-judging voice, any 'doom and gloom' and 'what if' thoughts, or any imagery that comes naturally to you in this situation. When you are aware of what these are, choose to be kind to yourself. Remember that healthy thinking is a choice, so see if you can cast some doubt on the truthfulness of these negative thoughts. Are they fact or fiction? And most of all, are they helpful to you?

Step 4: Connect to your peaceful place anchor

Bring another level of peace to this by connecting to your peaceful place and using your anchor while bathing in the good feeling that you get when you think of the deeper truth of your heart. Stay here for a minute or so.

Step 5: Mental rehearsal

Distancing rehearsal

Now, imagine you are in a movie theatre and you are watching a movie of the situation that used to trigger you, but now you are seeing things from a distance, feeling detached, neutral, and objective.

Drain all negative feelings away as if they were the colour being drained out of the picture. Imagine you are watching yourself in black and white, a character in a movie, now able to face their old

fears. When you reach the end of the movie, close the curtain, and take yourself back to your peaceful place for a minute or so. When you feel very relaxed, ask yourself:
On a scale of 0-10, how confident do I feel about coping with this situation? Make a mental note of the number.
Repeat the above process a couple of times using the same situation before moving on to the next step.

Affective rehearsal

Now, go back to the situation that used to trigger you, but imagine you are stepping inside the movie and you are the character in the film going through the target situation from the beginning to the end, as if it's happening right now. Reconnect to your deeper truth or power statement from Audio Session 2, and bring with you both the calm of your peaceful place and the good feeling you get when you connect to your deeper truth. Rehearse what it would be like to be perfectly calm and peaceful in this situation while always reminding yourself of the deeper truth of your heart.
Imagine how you'd like to ideally feel, and imagine what it would be like to feel that way. Go through the situation from the beginning to the end, and practice what it would be like to feel calm and peaceful about every aspect of this situation. When you have done that, fade everything to black and take yourself to your peaceful place again. When you feel very relaxed, ask yourself:
On a scale from 0-10, how confident do I feel about coping with this situation? Make a mental note of the number.

Behavioural rehearsal

Now, repeat the above step, this time focussing on the way you'd like to act in that situation. What would it be like to behave in a confident way? See yourself walk, talk, breathe, and move in the way you would if you felt confident and sure of yourself. If you find this challenging think of someone you admire who would behave confidently in a similar situation. Imagine stepping into their shoes.

Be your own version of them. Keep reminding yourself of your deeper truth, and when you have reached the end of the movie, take yourself to your peaceful place once again. When you feel very relaxed ask yourself:
On a scale from 0-10, how confident do I feel about coping with this situation? Make a mental note of the number.

Cognitive rehearsal

Now, repeat the above step, this time focussing on your deeper truth or power statement. Think that statement over and over and repeat it to yourself. Imagine what it would be like to really accept that idea more deeply.
Bring it fully into the situation, and imagine talking to yourself in a way that would be helpful, encouraging, and kind. Again, go through the whole scene imagining handling things in a much more positive way, allowing the calm of your peaceful place and the good feeling elicited by your deeper truth to always inform what you imagine. Go through the whole scene from beginning to end, and when you have reached the end, fade it all to black and take yourself to your peaceful place. When you feel very relaxed, ask yourself:
On a scale from 0-10, how confident do I feel about coping with this situation? Make a mental note of the number.
Repeat the cognitive rehearsal up to three more times and note the number each time. Thank yourself for putting in the hard work, and come out of hypnosis.

Homework Session 3

Listen to the audio recording every day, starting with situation 1/10 until your level of confidence is as close to 10 as you can get it. Then, engage in that situation in the real world, and when you feel you can cope well with it, move to the next situation on the list (i.e. 2/10).

In the next two bonus sessions, I shall explore how to overcome trauma and fear of rejection. I shall start with an explanation of how trauma is encoded in the brain and how it affects our levels of anxiety. I will then explain what is needed to move past it so you can eliminate all obstacles to your performance success. If you have not suffered trauma, or you are not worried about being rejected, feel free to jump this section onto part IV.

Chapter 8

Understanding Trauma

In this chapter, I shall give a brief description of how trauma is processed by the amygdala, and how to overcome its negative effects so you are no longer a victim to negative past events that still have a detrimental effect on your life.

Pattern matching [9]

Once a situation has been encoded as a threat by the amygdala, similar situations that match the original one will be seen as a threat, too, and will set the alarm off, producing similar symptoms to the first one. This is pattern matching, as understood by Joe Griffin, co-creator with Ivan Tyrrell of Human Givens Psychology, and it is the basis of human learning.

Let me first illustrate what I mean with an example from my life:

I play drums and my cat hates them. Whenever I sit on my stool, she knows I am about to play, and becomes distressed. She starts meowing loudly and then darts out of the room as fast as she can. I don't have to touch the drums for her to respond like this. Even if I sit on my stool for a different reason and don't play, she will react in the same way.

Pattern matching is the process by which our emotional brain matches a current environmental stimulus with a pre-existing template which triggers an immediate and unconscious emotional response. My sitting on the stool is the activating agent which

---

[9] For an extensive discussion of this concept refer to "Uncommon Psychotherapy" by Mark Tyrrell

matches my cat's memory of distress, which in turn makes her run out of the room.

In the case of fear, our limbic brain recognises a current stimulus as matching another one previously encoded as a threat. When this happens, the alarm goes on and it triggers the fear response. If you were robbed by a guy with a grey hoodie and this event traumatised you, now, whenever you see someone wearing a grey hoodie, you will respond with fear, even if the new person is harmless. This is because the hoodie has become a metaphorical symbol for the experience of being robbed.

This also works with attraction or other emotions triggered by specific stimuli. It's as if there were a 'tag' attached to the stimuli, encoding them as pleasant or unpleasant. This tag in turn activates an emotional response when other stimuli are recognised as similar to the ones already tagged.

For example, one of the boyfriends I had in my life was very tall and thin with curly blond hair. I was very much in love with him, and after the relationship was over, I continued being attracted to similar-looking men, even if they were completely different to my ex-boyfriend, or not right for me in all sorts of ways. Since pattern matching is a subconscious response to outside triggers, the activating agent was seeing a man who fit my visual pattern of attractiveness and the emotional response was that I felt attracted to him. Only later would I recognise that my feelings for that person had been based on an automatic response.

Of course, some pattern matches are hard wired, such as certain environmental triggers. For example, sand flying toward my eyes in a storm would trigger my template to protect them and I would respond by automatically blinking.

Pattern matching is the basis for all our physical processes, but because this system is sloppy, it can often give us faulty or incorrect responses. Our brains need to respond to all the challenges we face fast so we can stay safe. This means that we need to be able to anticipate possible dangers as quickly as we can, even at the cost of accuracy.

Erring on the side of caution is more effective for our survival than being accurate. So, for example, it would be better for our safety to respond to a hosepipe as if it were a dangerous snake than to take our time poking it with a stick it to see if it was indeed a real threat. The problem with this is that when a faulty pattern match takes hold, and the more the behaviour associated with it is repeated, the stronger the association becomes, because repetition strengthens neural pathways. This is the process known as "Hebbian Learning"—cells that fire together, wire together.

So, for example, if you had a bad experience with a music teacher who shouted at you every time you made a mistake at rehearsal, you may feel nervous and try to avoid making mistakes whenever you rehearse. In turn, this would make you tense and would most likely produce the very effect you were trying to avoid.

Or perhaps you raised your hand at school assembly when you were sixteen, but when you reached the microphone, your throat clenched and you felt terribly embarrassed. Now, every time it's your turn to speak, you may have the same symptoms and go blank. The more this happens, the more you expect it to happen, which primes you to respond the same way the next time.

Post-Traumatic Stress Disorder is a very extreme example of pattern matching in which the memory of the traumatic event has become locked in the amygdala. Whenever the memory is recalled, it is processed again as if it was a present emergency, and the person goes into fight or flight mode. When this happens repeatedly, the constant activation of the fight or flight response creates associations to even vague environmental stimuli that match the original trauma, which can lead to flashbacks and nightmares.

So, are we just victims to pattern matches? After all, our neocortex—our 'thinking' brain—is the new kid on the block compared to our emotional brain, evolutionarily speaking, and although we can reflect on and partially transcend our survival-geared pattern matching, our older emotional brain will always win in a match.

If we look at the person with PTSD, the extreme reaction of fear they experience will persist until they learn to process the troubling memory and transform it into a narrative. This is because while the memory remains 'live', the amygdala will be involved. Once it becomes something that happened in the past, the emotional reaction will diminish. For this to be possible, the person needs to learn to detach from the events as if they were observing themselves experiencing them from the outside.

Even if you don't have PTSD, if you have had trauma in your life and you still become upset when you think about it, you will need to learn to stand outside of yourself in order to interrupt the pattern match and transform it into a narrative.

How do you heal trauma?

To stop being triggered by the memories of your traumatic experiences, you need to return to the painful memories, but convince your amygdala that the danger is now over. The catch is that to do this successfully, you need to have the feelings connected to the original trauma activated. However, if you do arouse these feelings, the neocortex will shut down and no new information will be recorded.

To resolve this issue, you need to activate the traumatic memories, but also have a reliable method of switching off emotional arousal by systematically relaxing the body so that the cortex is still open to new information. In practice, this means that although you feel calm, the memories are still there.

Once this is achieved, you can relive the traumatic memory while keeping your emotional arousal down so you can feed new information into the cortex. This will change the meaning of the memory. The state of relaxation that you need for this process to work is induced through hypnosis, so that instead of simply reliving the disturbing traumatic memory from the inside, you can stand outside of it and therefore change your relationship to it.

This is something that is usually treated in a one on one session with any or a mix of the following procedures:

- Tony Robbins Scramble Technique[10]
- EFT[11]
- EMDR[12]
- Havening[13]
- Richard Bandler Dissociation Technique later developed by the Human Givens Institute into the Rewind technique[14]

I will include my version of these techniques in Bonus Audio Session 1, which you can listen to at your own discretion. For most people, it will be appropriate to listen to this session without a hypnotherapist present. However, if you feel you may not be able to remain calm during the process, I would suggest you skip it and contact a skilled hypnotherapist instead.

Although the practice itself can be reasonably quick and easy, it is important you don't re-traumatise yourself by simply reliving the trauma. If you need extra support, the therapist will be there with you to assist you so you are always in control and can stay calm throughout the process.

If you have experienced a trauma related to performing, it is important to address and dealt with it. A trauma is anything that is experienced as such. If something happened to you which, at the time, caused a deeply distressing emotion that overwhelmed your ability to cope, diminished your sense of self, or your ability to feel a full range of emotions, you experienced trauma.

---

[10] You can find this technique explained in the book by Tony Robbins "Awaken the Giant Within" p133

[11] EFT stands for Emotional Freedom Technique as described by Gary Craig in his book "EFT Handbook". For more practical information on the EFT points go to https://hypnotichealing.co.uk/techniques/eft-emotional-freedom-technique/

[12] EMDR stands for Eye Movement Desensitization and Reprocessing developed by Francine Shapiro.

[13] Havening was developed by Ronald Ruden and popularised by Paul McKenna.

[14] For more information on this technique visit https://www.uncommon-knowledge.co.uk/training/online/rewind-technique.html

It doesn't matter if, when you think about those events now, it seems crazy for you to still be affected by them. That judgement isn't going to change how you feel. The kind of trauma I am addressing here is of course related to performance and Bonus Audio Session 1 is for those of you who still feel upset in the present when you think about those traumatic events.

Remember that nothing is too small. It could be that you remember a time at school when you were bullied, or made fun of, or laughed at in public because you made a mistake reading. It could be a harsh teacher punishing you for being too loud, or for not speaking up. It could be being forced to say or do something in public that ended up in embarrassment. The possibilities are endless.

The good news is that it doesn't matter what the content of the trauma is, because the way we are going to deal with it is applicable to all kinds of traumatic events. So, if you think you experienced trauma around performing, I would urge you to either see a hypnotherapist and ask for trauma treatment or, if you feel you can remain calm while revisiting the event, try listening to Bonus Audio Session 1.

Bonus Session 1

Dealing with Traumatic Memories Safely

People often think trauma must be something big and dramatic. The truth is, you could have been traumatised by certain events in life whether they may seem small to someone else or if they happened a long time ago. One way of knowing whether you have any unresolved or unprocessed trauma, is to ask yourself the following questions:

1. *Did anything, for instance anything especially upsetting, happen before or around the time the first symptoms of performance anxiety began?*
2. *Does that memory still hurt? Is it upsetting to talk or think about it even now?*
3. *Does the memory feel more recent than it should, considering how long ago the event occurred? Does it feel like time has stood still?*
4. *Do even nebulous reminders set off flashbacks?*

If you answer yes to any of the above, you may suffer from unresolved trauma.

In this session, I will ask you to think of the memory that triggers the most anxiety or upset. It could be an embarrassing moment at work when you made a mistake, or it may be a parent shouting at you, or something more severe. After this exercise, you will either not have this memory, or it will be fuzzy. You may feel as if you are looking at it from a distance, or it may be there, but the peripheral details will be clearer and you will feel more objective and detached from it.

IMPORTANT:

Please note: this session is quite dynamic, and I would recommend you listen to the hypnotic audio rather than try to take yourself through it on your own, as that may be very challenging, if not impossible. Remember that you are in control. If at any time you feel upset, stop, take yourself to your peaceful place, and begin again only when you feel calm and peaceful.

It is now time to listen to your transformational hypnotic audio recording.

To do so, download the bonus package by typing the following link on your browser: https://tinyurl.com/daretobeseenonlinecourse

Here is a summary of the online content:

Step 1: Connect to the memory

Think about the disturbing memory, the most persistent memory that brings on the anxiety. Bring it back with as much detail as you can, and as much emotion as you experienced then.

Now, measure your level of discomfort when you think of it. On a scale of 0-10, how strong is the discomfort? Write this number down.

Step 2: EMDR rapid eye movement

Now, open your eyes, but keep your head still. Move your eyes on a horizontal line from left to right and then again to the left while thinking of the memory. Breathe deeply and repeat this at least 10 times while thinking of the disturbing memory. Notice any changes in your perception of the memory as you do so.

Step 3: Induce light hypnosis

Count backwards aloud from 30 to 0 by 3, like this: 30, 27, 24…
Count backwards from 40 by 4 aloud, slowly.
Induce hypnosis using an induction of your choice.

Step 4: Take yourself to your peaceful place

See Audio Session 1 for instructions.

Step 5: Connect to your inner strength.

Bring into your consciousness your Inner Teacher, your Higher Self, your Warrior, or Wise Woman / Man archetype. If you are religious, you can use God, or if you believe in Angels, bring them in. Invite whoever you feel safe with and protected by. To connect with your sense of inner strength, think of a time when you overcame an obstacle unexpectedly. Remember that inner voice that helped you through and guided your way.

Step 6: Rewind, scramble, reprocess

Imagine the traumatic events are like a movie with a beginning, a middle, and an end. The beginning is the point of safety before anything traumatic occurred. The end is when you are safe again and when everything is back to relative normality. Imagine you are sitting on your sofa and you have a remote control in your hand. You are now going to review the traumatic events backwards from the end to the beginning quickly, as if you were rewinding a VHS or DVD rapidly.

While you rewind the tape, place your hands on your arms in a cross shape and begin stroking the side of your arms in a downward motion.

When you reach the beginning of the tape, stop. Now, fast forward while imagining that you are walking with me on a beach. With each footstep you take in the sand, start counting aloud from 1 to 20. Keep stroking your arms down while you count. The idea is to self soothe, so keep doing this softly.

When you reach the end of the tape, stop, and hum the 'Happy Birthday Song' (or any childhood song that is associated with happy memories).

Now, repeat aloud:

I choose to let it go. It's in the past. It's safe to let it go.

Step 7: Check in and repeat

Check in with yourself. How much discomfort do you feel on a scale of 0 to 10 when you think of the initial memory?

Repeat the rewinding process at least three times or until the level of discomfort reaches 0 or as close to it as possible.

Step 8: Break your state and review your future.

When you reach the end, recite your phone number backwards. This will help you to come back to the present and break your state. Finally, review what your future is likely to look like now that the trauma has lost its power.

Step 9: Exit hypnosis.

When you are done, count yourself out of hypnosis by imagining you are going up a flight of stairs. When you reach the count of 5, you are back to your full conscious awareness.

You don't have to listen to this audio more than once. Only repeat it as much as you need to get as close to 0 as you can on your discomfort scale.

Bonus Session 2

Letting Go of Fear of Rejection

We are wired to take rejection seriously. Humans are social animals and their capacity to survive depends entirely on support from society. The ancestral part of our mind can be under the impression that if a person doesn't like us, this might mean we will be thrown out of the 'tribe' into the wilderness to fend for ourselves. In the past, this would have meant certain death. As a result, it is normal for us to be worried about not conforming or not being like others, and our minds try to protect us from danger by using anxiety as a preventative measure. But the truth is that we are a lot safer now than we have ever been because there are numerous 'tribes' within the fabric of society, so even if we don't fit into one, we will fit into another.

Society itself has also made big steps towards social inclusion and overall, we are all part of the human tribe. However, it can be hard to feel a sense of belonging when we have had experiences of being ostracised and left out in the past. Whether there have been times you felt rejected or whether you simply have a fear of not belonging, this will stand in your way of being comfortable with being seen, because you will be equating it with danger of expulsion. As humans, we learn from our experiences and tend to internalise judgement. If we have been harshly criticised in the past, we will tend to become our own worst critic. When we are rejected, we tend to reject ourselves. To negate this, we need to identify the episodes that caused these initial rejections and reframe them in a way that will allow us to let them go and replace self-rejection with self-acceptance.

With this in mind, it is time to listen to your transformational hypnotic audio recording.

IMPORTANT: Please note, this session is quite dynamic and I would recommend you listen to the hypnotic audio rather than try to take yourself through it on your own, as that may be very challenging if not impossible.

To do so, download the bonus package by typing the following link on your browser: https://tinyurl.com/daretobeseenonlinecourse

Here is a summary of the online content:

Step 1: Relax

Use an induction of your choice.

Step 2: Connect to the feeling of rejection, judgement and criticism

Recall the last time you felt rejected, judged, or criticised. Remember the last time you felt as though you did not belong. Imagine that scene again. Amplify that feeling. Imagine you could turn the intensity up, as if turning a dial all the way to the right. Now, go back to the first time you remember experiencing this feeling. If you get a clear idea, skip to step 5.

Step 3: Regression to childhood home

Otherwise, imagine going back in time to your childhood home. See yourself going inside your bedroom and meeting your younger self there. She or he will know who you are and will be perfectly comfortable with you.

Step 4: Exploratory dialogue with your inner child.

Ask your younger self a series of questions:
- *Are you happy or unhappy?*
- *Who loves you?*
- *Do you feel loveable?*
- *What do the people raising you do or not do that make you feel unloved?*
- *Who is rejecting you?*
- *What are the people around you doing or not doing that make you feel rejected?*

Step 5: Explore scenes where you felt rejection

See yourself in a scene that has something to do with when and how you first acquired this perception that people might be rejecting you. Allow a scene that has something to do with the feeling that you are not good enough to emerge. Imagine you are in a time tunnel that pulls you back to a vivid, vital scene that is the cause, the reason, the root of your fear of rejection. Be there and experience it as if it's happening now. Describe what you hear and see in the present tense.
- *Are you inside or outside?*
- *Is it day or night?*
- *Are you alone or with others?*
- *How old do you feel?*
- *What are you doing, seeing, feeling?*
- *What are you experiencing?*
- *What are you hearing that is being said about you, to you, or around you?*
- *What's going on?*

Pay special attention to how you feel. Be aware of what you are experiencing as if it happened yesterday. When you have finished exploring this scene, imagine putting it inside your left hand as if it were a scene of a moment in your past you were watching on a DVD. Now, connect to a different scene that has to do with a similar feeling of not being good enough.

Allow another scene that relates to how, when, where, and why you acquired this fear and belief that people will reject you. Repeat the process above and notice what you are feeling. When you have finished exploring this second scene, put it in your left hand and repeat the process with a third scene.

Step 6: Reframe these scenes

When you are done exploring the three scenes relating to how and why you were rejected, imagine that you are holding a DVD that contains all of them in your left hand. At the same time, picture holding a DVD of a scene from today in your right hand. In the scene, this very issue is holding back from what you want to do. As you look at the scenes in your left hand, let your brilliant mind understand exactly how and where and why you have acquired this fear of being rejected. Find the connection, the common theme that holds them together.

Perhaps bullies at school said really mean things to you and you concluded they were right. Perhaps your parents preferred your brother or sister over you and you took it to mean your siblings were better than you. Perhaps your teacher liked all the other kids, but shouted at you and as a consequence you started believing your were ugly, stupid, poor, or different. Begin to see how and why you acquired these beliefs. As you do, your subconscious mind is becoming aware that you formed misconceptions about yourself because of these events.

You came to conclusions about yourself and formed beliefs based on these experiences when you were too little to understand what was really going on. You formed opinions about yourself that were based on events that had little to do with you and a lot to do with the others around you. You came to the conclusion that people would reject you, that you are not good enough, and that you don't measure up to others. But now you are an adult and you understand so much more.

And understanding is power. And as you look through these scenes again, this understanding is so powerful, liberating, and transforming because you understand why and how those scenes affected you, but you also understand something else: that you're not that little kid anymore. You understand that it will never ever again for the rest of your life be relevant or necessary or appropriate or even remotely interesting for you to feel those feelings ever again.

So now, cement this understanding by saying aloud:

I am not that kid because… and complete the sentence.

That's not me because… (i.e. I am an adult and I know now I am worthy of love and belonging)

Repeat this process until you are satisfied.

Step 7: Upgrade the child and become a loving parent to yourself

It is time now to go back to your childhood home where you met your younger self. Wrap your arms around that child or take her by the hand. Take her back to where you live now. Show her how different her life is going to be from now on. You are now going to take care of her the way she always wished someone would care for her.

Remember all the things that you most wanted to hear as a child and tell those things to your child.

For example: *You're a great kid. I love you. I am so lucky to be your mum/dad. I am so blessed to raise a kid as great as you. You're so sweet. You're gorgeous. You're intelligent. You're loveable. When you grow up, you're going to find so many people that love you because you are loveable. You're a good kid. I'm glad you're alive. I'm glad you're a boy/girl. I'm glad you are you.*

Add the words that you most needed to hear as a child. Repeat them aloud while holding your child close.

If relevant, consider adding the following sentences:

- *I'm becoming a loving parent to you.*
- *No one in the world can play this role like I can.*
- *I love you exactly the way you are.*
- *I love you completely and unconditionally.*
- *You never ever have to earn my love.*
- *You're safe with me.*
- *I'm here protecting you always.*
- *I'll always have time for you.*
- *I will always listen to you.*
- *Together there is nothing we can't do.*

Even if you feel that your parents didn't love you or want you, remember that the universe wanted you to be here. You are a gift to your parents and you are meant to be on this earth. And even if they failed to honour you, the universe wanted you to be here and it wanted you to be you. There is nobody in the world who is exactly like you and there will never be another you. The universe that put you on this planet will support you a hundred percent.

Step 8: Reframe critical people and praise yourself

Remember that nobody can reject you unless you let them. Critical people have the most criticism reserved for themselves. They're unhappy. They don't like themselves and they criticise everyone else, too, so that other people will feel as bad as they feel. Superior people, on the other hand, praise others and you are becoming an expert at praising yourself. Choose to praise yourself from now on by saying to yourself, "I'm lovable. I love myself. I accept myself. I believe in myself. I'm here with something valuable to offer."

And as you praise yourself every day, your self-esteem will increase. As it does, so will your sense of self-worth. And when your sense of self-worth goes up, so will other people's sense of your worth and value.

Remember that nobody can reject you unless you give them your permission. And from now on, tell yourself that you choose to never do that again, because you know the truth about yourself. And the truth about you is that you matter. You are significant. You belong.

Step 9: Let go of old beliefs

See all those outdated beliefs shrinking and disappearing. See all that contributed to your negative beliefs, your misconceptions about yourself being shattered and smashed, eradicated. See those beliefs that you used to carry around out of your life, in the past, behind you.

Step 10: Rewrite the scenes

Now, go back to the three scenes and re-write the endings the way you would have wanted them to be.
Perhaps the person who bullied you before, now wants to hang out with you and be your friend. Perhaps you now stand up for yourself. Maybe you laugh it all off because you see how the person that hurt you was hurting too. Hurting others is often a way for people to find a way out of their pain. Or maybe the parents that used to that put you down, suddenly realise what a great kid you are. When you change these scenes, you empower yourself, so make them look the way you would have liked them to be. This will create a powerful transformation within you, because your mind believes what you tell it.

Step 11: Come out of hypnosis

When you are ready, come out of hypnosis by counting from 1-5 and imagining you are going up a flight of stairs. This session can be very emotionally draining and intense, so you may feel tired for a few hours or even days afterwards. This is a good sign, so just rest up and be gentle with yourself.

Only listen to this session once.

Homework Bonus Session 2

Look at the mirror and say to yourself, "I am enough". If any objections come up, write them down. Then pretend you are in a court of law and you are the defendant lawyer.

Write down the objection to that objection and keep going until there are no more objections.

For example:

Affirmation: *I am enough.*

Objection: *No, you're not. You are lazy. You never finish what you start.*

Objection to the Objection: *That is not true. I finished school. I completed all my assignments and passed my exams. I didn't finish the university course I started because it was not the right course for me.*

Practice praising yourself daily. Pat yourself on the back, and celebrate every little success. Make yourself feel good about the effort you are putting into projects. Focus on efforts rather than results.

Congratulations. You have now finished part II of this course. In part III, we will be focussing on leaving behind toxic habits and creating a new you that is anxiety free and lives in the now. This will allow you to really be present during presentations, speeches, interviews, auditions, or concerts. This is important, because only when you are present in the moment, you can truly give your best.

PART III—
SESSIONS 4—7

CREATING A NEW YOU

DOWNLOAD the Dare to Be Seen
BONUS PACKAGE

including a

FREE AUDIOBOOK,
CHECKLIST and WORKBOOK

Templates, Training, Resources to Kickstart your Journey
into Authentic Confidence under the Spotlight!

TO DOWNLOAD GO TO
https://hypnotichealing.co.uk/bonuses

Chapter 9

Are you a Victim
of Conditioning?

You are who you were conditioned to be

In this chapter, I am going to talk about how negative past
experiences can shape our identity and how to transcend this
negative programming to create a better future for ourselves.
To become the best version of ourselves we could possibly be, we
need to first understand what made us who we are today. Of
course, we are all a mix of nurture and nature, and our behaviour is
a result of our genetic makeup as well as our education. But apart
from genetic tendencies, how do external factors impact how we
develop psychologically and therefore, who we become as adults?
I believe all of us follow a 'script' which is based on often
unconscious ideas we have about ourselves. These form our identity
and the beliefs we have about the world. In other words, we don't
see reality as it is, but as *we are*.
So, how do we form these ideas? How is the script written? I
believe the answer is: "through conditioning".

What is conditioning?

Conditioning means
    1. To have a significant influence on or determine the
        outcome of something.
    2. To train to behave in a certain way.

Let's unpack this. When I think of conditioning, I think of the
conditions by which something is included or excluded from the

idea of what we consider to be our identity and our concept of reality. These conditions act as a filter through which certain aspects and qualities of ourselves are accepted or rejected as desirable or undesirable.

The conditions are based on value judgements that define what is good, bad, true, false, beautiful, ugly, right, or wrong. In other words, these judgements create beliefs about how knowledge can be acquired, what constitutes truth, what is ethical, and what is aesthetically pleasing. So, how are these value judgements formed? When we are young children, we are free and uninhibited. We are a clean slate. We are born with some innate tendencies that we inherit from our parents and the way we express our needs depends on those tendencies. However, as babies, we express our needs and wants without filters. If we are hungry, we cry for attention. If we feel affection, we freely express it. If we want to jump up and down out of excitement, we do it. That is, until somebody tells us off for it.

Throughout childhood, we are progressively trained to welcome certain behaviours as desirable and reject others as not. This is done by having love withdrawn when we exhibit behaviours that are not approved by our caregivers, peers, or society at large.

Children depend entirely on the support and approval of their caregivers for both their emotional and material needs. This goes beyond just parents and includes all the significant influences that are present in a child's world. When a caretaker or important person in a child's life disapproves of the child's behaviour, this is experienced as a very serious threat by that child.

This is because children can't see the difference between their behaviour being disapproved of and themselves being rejected. If approval is withdrawn, the child could suffer serious consequences. The message is that their life support may be withdrawn if they don't behave or act in a certain way.

Let me illustrate this with a made-up scenario:

Let's assume Tim is 6 years old when his father comes to pick him up from school. That day, Tim is upset because his school mate, Dave, called him names in front of his friends. Tim explains to his father that he has failed to retaliate and in fact, he was humiliated in front of the other children.

While telling the story to his dad, Tim starts to cry. This seems to trigger his father. Perhaps he is reminded of himself when he, too, was bullied as a kid and was never able to resolve his own feelings of inadequacy thereafter. In a misguided attempt at saving his own son from suffering a similar fate, instead of reassuring him, he tells him to "stop whining" because boys don't cry.

He also tells Tim to just hit the other boy harder. Hearing this, his son learns that crying is wrong and a sign of weakness. He feels shame whenever tears well up in his eyes and he grows up unable to show vulnerability. He learns that violence is the best way to win respect. From then on, he starts to hide his feelings and makes fun of anyone who doesn't do the same.

From this example, it is clear how Tim accepted his father's dysfunctional beliefs as his own and created his self-image, goals, and code of conduct based on them. In other words, he was conditioned to behave in ways that might not serve his best interests and that did not necessarily correspond to his natural inclinations.

This happens to all of us as children, because until adulthood, our brains are like sponges; they need to absorb as much information as they can in as little time as possible to have the best shot at survival. The critical faculty is something that needs to be trained and cultivated and often, this does not occur until at least our teenage years.

The most important need for a child is attention and approval. Children learn by imitating the behaviours they see around them. They keenly observe the feedback they receive when they exhibit those behaviours themselves. If they are punished for them, they usually avoid them. However, in cases of neglect, they may opt to imitate behaviours that are frowned upon which, nevertheless, get them attention. This is because there is only one thing worse than being punished, and that is being ignored.

As children, we adopt those behaviours as our own and we also form our sense of identity based on what we perceive to be the

judgement of others on our character. Statements such as, "You are just as clever as uncle John..." or "You'll never amount to anything" can become powerful messages that will shape who we become.
I like to think of the mind as a complex computer that comes with basic hardware. The hardware is the genes we inherit from our parents, the building blocks that constitute the foundations of who we are; in other words, our nature. However, it is the operating system—the software—that makes a computer work in a particular way. This is written throughout our lives and it is based on experience.
This 'software' script will shape a person's entire life if left unchallenged. It's an unconscious map that depicts the version of who you believe yourself to be and directs you to live a specific kind of life, influencing outcomes such as your self-esteem, your status in society, your level of accomplishment, and even the status of your relationships.
If the significant others in your early life were critical or negative on a regular basis, or if your experiences were particularly negative or traumatic, this could easily lead you to internalise that critical voice and develop negative core beliefs that will limit your growing into a well-rounded, multifaceted individual.
You could become an adult with a small identity, believing you are not good enough, not worthy of being seen and heard, not worthy of love and acceptance, not worthy of belonging, and therefore, headed for a life of broken hopes, broken relationships, and broken dreams.
Carrying such a damaged sense of self is too painful to bear without some sort of 'medicine'. As a result, you might develop coping mechanisms such as anxiety, addiction, or the impossible search for perfectionism.

Are we all just victims of conditioning?

So, are we all just victims of conditioning? Or can we overcome it and become conscious creators of our own destiny? To find the answer, let's look at the father of 'classical conditioning', Ivan Pavlov.

Ivan Pavlov was a Russian physiologist who taught dogs to respond with salivation to a trigger, such as the ring of a bell. Every time he rang the bell, food would appear and the dogs would salivate. However, after adequate repetitions, the dogs would salivate even if the food was not present, because a powerful association had been created between the ringing of the bell and the dispensation of food.

Many of us are like Pavlov's dogs. The bell is the trigger behaviour that we have learned to associate with the reward we seek (such as approval) and we keep repeating this behaviour even when we don't receive the reward. Alternatively, we avoid a certain situation that we have associated with danger, even if the danger has long gone. We just live our lives on autopilot. We follow the script that was written in the past, and that's that. We say: 'this is who I am, I cannot help it'.

Let's look at this in practice. Let's suppose Luke is a creative and off-beat child with unappreciative parents. The latter have high-powered careers and are often highly strung when coming home from work. They value conformity and obedience and feel threatened by his 'weird' and original ways. So, whenever they feel he is 'too much' for them, they ridicule and shame him. Luke feels unloved, not accepted for who he is and tries various ways out. First, he may become angry and may try to rebel, but his parents just label him as 'naughty' and out of control. His father gives him the silent treatment until he apologises and complies with his demands. Luke cannot stay his ground and eventually, caves in. He starts pretending to adopt the identity his father expects of him, playing the role of the 'good boy' but actually cutting himself off from his authentic self.

Years later, Luke seems to have become a shy guy, unassuming and not very good at being assertive. After spending his childhood escaping into the world of fiction, he has developed an ability for writing great characters, but after one of his books is awarded a prize and his career starts to go somewhere, he is asked to give presentations and do book tours. He wants to share the fruits of his creative self, but being on stage terrifies him.

This is because, although Luke longs to be authentic, doing so is matched with danger. Authenticity is associated with punishment and shame, and therefore, very threatening. In Luke's case, being shy is not a 'natural' and unchanging personality trait, but a result of his conditioning. Should he simply accept this as his destiny, or could he change?

The difference between we humans—you, me, and Luke—and Pavlov's dogs is that we have self-awareness. And with self-awareness comes the power of choice. It is up to us whether we want to succumb to our 'fate' and follow the script we have been handed, or not.

When we become aware of our specific conditioning, we have a choice. We can be victims or victors. We can choose whether to feel sorry for ourselves and blame our parents, teachers, and abusers for who we are today, or we can choose to move away from victim mentality. If we realise we are not our past, we can turn it into wisdom. If we take responsibility for who we are today, we can create a different future for ourselves. We can allow our tormentors to continue to have power over us, or we can choose to take our power back. The choice is entirely in our own hands.

If we decide to exercise our free will, we can recognise the pattern matches and associations that keep us stuck in our old ways. We can do the work and save ourselves. We can use our power of choice to recondition ourselves. We, unlike a bug-ridden computer, can rewrite our own software, fix the buggy script, and write a wonderfully epic ending to our story.

In the next chapter, we shall take a closer look at how to use the LAMA Method to let go of our faulty conditioning so we can create a better future for ourselves.

Chapter 10

How to Recondition Yourself with the LAMA Method

In this chapter, I will explain how to use the LAMA method to let go of old, unwanted behaviours so you can create a new version of yourself on stage and beyond.

Change your ways through self-directed neuroplasticity

Every time you repeat a certain behaviour in response to a trigger, neurons fire together and wire together, creating neural pathways. Each time the behaviour is repeated, the corresponding neural pathways are reinforced. On the other hand, when you do not engage in that specific behaviour for long enough, the neural pathways associated with it start to weaken. You may have heard of the phrase 'use it or lose it'. Effectively, the brain has limited space and optimises it by allowing the survival of only the busiest synapses.

To illustrate how this works, let me give you an example. I was a Latin and Greek A-student at high school. However, I do not have much recall of these languages any more. Twenty years have passed and I have not practiced them since. As a result of not using my skills in this area, I lost them.

When you use your attention deliberately to make a new choice, the anterior cingulate cortex is activated and this leads to lasting changes in behaviour. Imagine you are in a snowy forest. You have walked down a certain path on many occasions and therefore, you know it very well. Even though this track may not be particularly interesting, it is easy to follow because it feels familiar and well-trodden.

You could continue to go down this path for the rest of your life, but one day, you get the idea that maybe you could clear the way and walk in a different direction. At first, it doesn't look easy, but you decide to try. After some effort to clear the terrain from snow, you are pleasantly surprised to find the new path ends up near a beautiful lake.

If tomorrow, you came back to the spot where you started the journey, you would have a new choice; you could follow the old path which is still familiar and mostly clear of snow, or you could take the new one. Remembering your preferred destination would help you decide which path to choose.

Now, if every time you kept choosing the new path, eventually, it would become well-trodden and more familiar while the original one would soon be covered in snow. In this analogy, walking down the old path represents the familiar response to a stimulus that is the old behaviour, while making a new trail represents behaving in a way that is different from what you are used to.

Attention is like a vacuum cleaner

The mind takes the shape of what it rests upon, and the brain takes the shape of what the mind is fixed on. The latter is really just a flow of information which we can choose to either leave undirected, or to consciously direct using our attention.

If we focus on gratitude and self-appreciation, for example, the brain will shape itself to support greater resilience and happiness. On the other hand, if we focus on resentment and self-criticism, the brain will respond with low mood and irritability.

In the same fashion, when we focus our attention on how worried we are about making mistakes during a presentation, we will prime ourselves to be nervous and do poorly as a result. Alternatively, if we fix on having fun and being able to cope no matter what, we will prime ourselves to do much better.

Attention is like a vacuum cleaner. Whatever you focus on is sucked into the brain. So, you must train it to rest on what's useful through concentration. This is what I call self-directed neuroplasticity, which is what happens when we use self-hypnosis. If you want to know more about it, I strongly recommend you read the book by Norman Doidge, *The Brain That Changes Itself.*

The mind is a garden

So, how does this work exactly? Think of the mind as a garden. Whatever you feed, grows. It is up to you whether to feed the weeds or the apple tree. If you want the latter to grow, stop watering the weeds and start tending to your tree every day. However, remember that the ground needs to be prepared properly before you even plant the seed. An adequate amount of water and sun needs to be provided for its needs. Then you will need to wait and return to it every day, keeping up the work patiently and consistently.

If you just tend your garden sporadically, you won't get the results you want. The seed, which is very fragile at first, needs tender care. Only repetition is going to ensure that the seed has enough strength to develop into a sapling and eventually into a beautiful tree.

In the same way, if you want to reprogram your mind with good, healthy thoughts and habits, you need to know how to effectively nurture them by offering them your attention patiently, consistently, and repeatedly.

In our minds, just like in a garden, whatever you feed grows and whatever you don't nurture dies. Our brain is plastic. It changes constantly. What we don't use we lose, and what we focus on expands. So, let's start pulling weeds and plant flowers in the gardens of our mind.

Where attention goes, energy flows; so let's repeat our new behaviours and thoughts and let us reward ourselves when we do things right. The best way to do so is to repeatedly direct our conscious attention to where we want our inner tree to grow. This offers the best rewards when done in hypnosis.

How to learn better behaviours

Learning is all about selecting and prioritising information we consider important. Reconditioning means replacing old learning with new and better learning.

This process follows four stages:

- Becoming aware of unconsciously familiar dysfunctional behaviours;
- Choosing to adopt new functional behaviours;
- Replacing the old behaviours with new ones;
- Making the new behaviours unconsciously familiar.

This is possible with the help of transformational hypnotherapy. To understand how this works, consider the three main ways in which we learn, namely through:

- emotionally intense experiences
- repetition of experiences
- mental rehearsal

Emotionally intense experiences

We interpret emotionally intense experiences by giving them a positive or negative meaning. These meanings inform our beliefs about life and ourselves. When they are highly positive, we label the events as 'peak' and when they are highly negative, we see them as 'traumatic'.

For example, if we are attacked by a dog and experience intense fear or physical damage, we may form the belief that all dogs are dangerous. On the other hand, if we feel extreme elation after winning a swimming competition, we may form the belief not only that swimming is the best sport, but that we are excellent swimmers.

Hypnosis can help us reconnect with powerful peak experiences and elicit intense new ones. By using it in this way, we can form new positive unconscious beliefs that stick.

Repetition

Repetition is another powerful learning tool. This could apply to an activity we repeatedly engage in, as in when we hone a skill. For example, if we practice guitar over and over, eventually, we will become unconsciously skilled at the instrument and believe we are competent players.

Repetition is also responsible for us learning beliefs about ourselves, whether they reflect the truth or not. If we repeatedly receive criticism, for example, we'll tend to believe it is true. So, if we are told repeatedly that we are inept, we may come to believe we are stupid and act accordingly.

Through repetition, what was once conscious effort, becomes unconscious competence. Take driving, for example; at first, we may have to concentrate hard to learn a variety of actions that can feel overwhelming. But by repeating them, we eventually drive without thinking about it. When this happens, it means the autonomic nervous system[15] is now taking care of the behaviour automatically. This is how habits are formed.

By repeating positive suggestions during hypnosis, we can accept new helpful beliefs about ourselves, which in turn, will help us perform better. By repeating these positive hypnotic processes, we can cement the new beliefs until they become part of who we are.

Mental rehearsal

The third and less known way of learning, which is very relevant to us, is through virtual practice. When we practice something solely in the imagination, this is called mental rehearsal.

Since hypnosis is a natural state of relaxation, inward focus, and high concentration, it is optimal for learning new behaviours.

---

[15] The part of the nervous system responsible for control of the bodily functions not consciously directed, such as breathing, the heartbeat, and digestive processes.

Spending time in hypnosis mentally rehearsing the type of behaviour, thoughts, and feelings we want, is almost as good as having an experience that will elicit them in the real world.

This works because the brain doesn't differentiate between what you imagine doing and what you really do. Have you ever had a dream that someone you loved died and it caused you to wake up crying? Or have you ever thought about eating your favourite food and found that you were salivating? Have you ever noticed that when you repetitively imagine anxiety-provoking events taking place, you can experience physical symptoms such as nausea, diarrhoea, or a constant need to pee?

This is because your mind responds to what you imagine, whether it is real or not. Imagining a threat for long enough will trigger the fight or flight response, even if the threat is not real. When that happens, your sympathetic nervous system will be activated and stress chemicals will be released, causing all sorts of symptoms. (I describe this in detail in Audio Session 1 and Chapter 8.)

Mental rehearsal is very powerful, and it works in the positive just as well as in the negative. Every time we use mental rehearsal in an emotionally and cognitively beneficial way, we reinforce the neural pathways associated with that behaviour.

This is best illustrated by some studies in which subjects were put inside an MRI scanner and were asked to practice scales with a real instrument versus imagining doing so. Amazingly, on both occasions, the same areas of the brain lit up. In terms of learning, the results were close too. The implication here is that learning 'in vitro' is almost as good as learning 'in vivo' and in fact, prepares you for the real thing. So, if you rehearse something mentally first, it is almost as good as if you really did it.

By virtually rehearsing the desired responses to a fearful trigger in an imagined scenario, you will have conditioned yourself to exhibit the desired responses more easily in real life. This is because virtual rehearsal creates the same neural pathways that would be created if you engaged in that behaviour in external reality. It's like theatre rehearsals; you learn how to act before the show happens, so on opening night, you are ready for the real thing.

To summarise, re-conditioning happens when we engage in an active effort to positively reshape our identity and behaviour while in a state of relaxation and concentration such as self-hypnosis. We do this by internalising emotionally intense positive experiences, letting go of negative ones, learning new ways of seeing ourselves, and reinforcing this new vision with repeated reminders over a period of time. This is what we will do using the LAMA Method.

Let go of the past and move ahead with the LAMA Method

LAMA stands for: let go and move ahead. Letting go of the past is a choice. If you want to create a better future, you need to let go of your familiar negative habits and replace them with better ones. The old, familiar worrying habit must go. The old familiar indulging in catastrophic 'what if' scenarios must stop. The old familiar habit of dwelling on all the terrible things that happened must be replaced by new, helpful habits.

We do this by accepting the past for what it is, sitting with any emotion that emerges, and allowing those emotions to be expressed so we can move forward. We then choose to keep the positive lessons we have learned from what has gone before so we can leave the rest behind. This allows us to replace negative meanings associated with past events with something more positive and helpful.

Then, we actively *choose new habits*. We choose to be present in the here and now. We create a better future by choosing the emotions we want in the present: calm, trust, and confidence in our ability to not only cope, but to thrive.

In the next four sessions, we shall engage in practices that will help you do that. You will let go of the past, taking with you only what serves you. You will let go of catastrophising. You will let go of worrying. And you will learn how to be present in the moment. This will help you remain relaxed on stage and perform at your very best in a way that you never thought possible before.

Audio Session 4

Letting Go of the Past

In this session, you will learn to honour the positives in your past and to carry them with you. You will discover how to appreciate the lessons you have learned from it and to leave behind everything else. You will then focus on creating the future that you want. You can use this session to let go of any negative situations that hold you back from being seen in all your glory.

The past always has something to teach us, but we often dwell only on its negative aspects. This is tantamount to looking at the bygone year only remembering the days of rain. Instead, we can take what we have learned from our experiences to create a better present. We need to remember that every day is an opportunity to break free from what has previously occurred so we can create a different reality.

The past is gone, but if we live in it, we throw away both our present and our future. It is like living in a dark room with the curtains drawn, forgetting that the sun is still shining outside. Or trying to catch the water that goes down the drain when you have a shower. The water is gone and can never come back.

It is now time to listen to your transformational hypnotic audio recording.

To do so, download the bonus package by typing the following link on your browser: https://tinyurl.com/daretobeseenonlinecourse

Alternatively, you can make up your own session. Begin by recording the induction and deepening as described in Chapter 6. Speak slowly and clearly into your recording device and record the following points before finishing with the "awakening" section also described in Chapter 6.

Here is a summary of the online content:

Step 1: Induce hypnosis

Use your favourite induction.

Step 2: Step on your timeline

Imagine you are standing in front of a line drawn in the sand. On the left of the line is the past. The middle of the line is the present, and the future is to the right of the line. Now, imagine you are standing in the middle. You are carrying a suitcase with you and you are about to go on a journey backwards in time. As you turn to face the past, imagine you see a house behind you; this is the house of all your past experiences. This house contains everything that has ever happened to you in relation to performing, giving presentations, auditions, interviews, or speeches. It contains all that has made you who you are today.

Step 3: The house of the past

Now, imagine stepping inside your house. You are going through all the rooms, collecting only the objects and memories that will be useful for you to bring with you from now on. Everything else will be left behind. Your suitcase is magical and can contain entire universes inside it. So, fill it with only the experiences that are helpful. Fill it with all the lessons that you have learnt from; the difficult situations you have lived through. When you are done, step out of the house and face it again with your suitcase in your hand.

Step 4: Letting go

Now that your suitcase contains everything you need from the past, it is time for you to destroy the house. Choose a way that feels satisfying. You could burn it down. You could call on a tsunami to wash it away. You could allow a tornado to shatter it into a million pieces. Be creative and make it work for you. When the house is gone, you are ready to turn ahead to the future and say goodbye to it forever.

Step 5: Envision the future

Now, as you face forward, it is time to envision your future. Visualise in as much detail as possible what you want your future to be like when it comes to performing. Imagine the perfect audition, interview, speech, or gig. Imagine yourself going through it in the way you want to. Imagine feeling the way you want to feel from now on in those circumstances: confident, calm, with all the self-belief you would ever need. Again, be creative, dwell on the good feelings you want to experience, and visualise going through the 'performance' from beginning to end in the perfect way for you.

Step 6: Exit hypnosis

Count yourself out of hypnosis in the usual way.
Listen to this recording until you feel you have thoroughly let go of the past. It may be that once is enough, or you may need to repeat the process several times.

Homework Session 4

1) Create a ritual around getting rid of your 'house of the past'

For example, you could draw a house on a piece of paper filled with objects and people that represent what you need to leave behind. Use colours that are meaningful to you and don't worry about being unable to draw. What is important is to connect with the symbols in the picture. Once you have drawn the house, get rid of it. You could literally burn the paper. You could bury it in your garden. You could draw a huge black cloud over it until you cannot see it anymore. If, on the other hand, you possess an object that reminds you of a negative experience connected to your anxiety, choose to deliberately destroy it in a ritual fashion. Your mind works with metaphors, so follow your instincts and trust your creativity.

2) Create a symbol representing a new future you

Your subconscious responds to symbols, so create a symbol that represents the self-belief, the calm, the enjoyment, and the confidence that you want to bring into your performances. Take that symbol with you and draw power from it before every performance.
For example, you could draw a picture that represents your new confident self and put it in your pocket before you go on stage, touching it every

time you need more confidence. Or, if there was a piece of music in your visualisation that made you feel powerful and happy, listen to it before your performances. Or, if you have a significant object, piece of jewellery, or piece of clothing that feels meaningfully connected to your hypnotic visualisation, wear it during your performances.

3) Look back at the present from the future

Imagine it's six months from now and you have achieved all of your performance goals. Look back over the past few months: what have you done that has made it possible for you to be here today? Stand up, get excited and talk about everything that has happened as if it was the best time of your life. Imagine you are telling your best friend about it. Time yourself and spend exactly five minutes doing this.

In the next chapter, we will focus on how to let go of catastrophic thinking so you can enjoy peace of mind in the days before your speech, audition, concert, or presentation.

Audio Session 5

Letting Go of 'What if'

In this chapter, we will explore why 'what if' thinking is so damaging and how to rob it of its influence so you feel empowered to cope, no matter what happens.

What if you forgot the words of your speech mid-sentence? What if you didn't know the answers at an interview? What if your hand trembled in the middle of an audition? What if you quoted the wrong information when presenting your project? What if you sang out of tune? It could happen, right? Sure, it could. But would it be as bad as you think?

The answer lies in the use of your imagination. Catastrophic thinking is a way of misusing your imagination to predict terrible consequences even to minor setbacks. You imagine something going wrong and then you feel sure a disaster would follow. But is this really accurate? And does it help?

First of all, the exaggerated scenario you are imagining in your head is not reality. It is fiction. But your brain doesn't know the difference, remember? And because of this, your body reacts to this fantasy as if it were real. As a result, you are more likely to panic and make the very scenario you are afraid of come true. Your mind is always listening, and what you focus on, you move towards. So, when you imagine the worst, you are effectively training your mind to get the very result you don't want.

So, what good does it do to indulge in imagining catastrophic scenarios? Does it stop them from happening? No. You could spend all your time imagining the worst. The wing of a plane could fall on your house and reduce it to nothing. But would imagining this in advance stop it from happening? I doubt it. So, why waste your time and make yourself miserable? The truth is 'what if thinking' not only doesn't help you, it makes things worse.

The best option you have when it comes to 'what ifs' is to make them your arch enemy. You could decide right now that the 'what ifs' are just a plain waste of your time. They do nothing for you, and in fact, they even ruin your present. But what if... you can't stop thinking that way? See, you did it again!

Seriously though, no matter what you do, when you repeat a behaviour enough times, it becomes your default mindset. It's so familiar that it seems natural. But remember, you always have a choice. You can walk down the path you always walk down, or you could change direction.

If, however, you choose to indulge in 'what ifs' for a little while longer, my invitation is to also choose to see yourself being able to cope regardless. Let's face it, even if the worst-case scenario happened in your life, you would find a way to cope. When it comes to it, we want to survive, and we are a lot more resilient than we give ourselves credit for.

Even if you lost your house, your job, and your partner—if you had enough of a desire to keep going, you would find a way to do so. Even if you had a stroke, you could learn how to talk again! So, you could certainly cope if you made a mistake and looked a bit silly on stage. Start telling yourself that, and you will begin to feel a lot better.

I'll give you an example. I once had a client who felt very insecure about blushing while giving a presentation. She used to worry that her audience would think she was unprofessional and she would feel so ashamed, it would be humiliating. Given she had a history of blushing in the "wrong" moment, it was certainly possible—even likely—that it would happen again. She had to change how she envisioned her way of reacting to that event.

I suggested that instead of imagining herself losing the plot, she would start reminding herself she could cope. It may not be ideal, but she would survive. This took the edge off, because it transformed her thinking from black and white into a greyscale. Instead of believing that the presentation would either work or be a disaster, she started framing it differently. Her self-talk transformed into: 'even if this doesn't work, I will survive and eventually, I'll be okay'.

The other reason why this reframe worked, is that it transformed a demand into a preference. Sure, it would be better if she delivered her speech perfectly, but making a mistake wouldn't be the end of the world either. When you stop demanding perfection, it takes the pressure off and it makes it easier to cope with the consequences of even the worst-case scenario.

So, remember, it is not the events, but rather the meaning you give those events that make you miserable (or happy). And what you expect tends to be realised. So, try to stop taking yourself so seriously and start laughing at the possibility that everything might go wrong. Say to yourself, "No matter what happens, I'll be ok". The answer to the "what ifs" is "so what? I'll cope!"

Preparatory exercises

If you find yourself overestimating the possibility that things will turn out badly, or if you often jump to worst case scenarios, you are probably looking at the world in a way that makes it seem more dangerous than it really is.

It's as if you are wearing the opposite of rose-tinted glasses. Your glasses are like the distorting mirrors you find in amusement park horror houses. You see every negative thought as a fact. You assume you have little ability to cope with life's problems and you discredit your positive qualities.

These irrational, pessimistic attitudes are known as cognitive distortions. Have a look at the following list and complete the exercise outlined underneath it after you have listened to the hypnotic session.

Cognitive distortions

All or nothing thinking—Looking at things in black or white categories with no middle ground.

e.g. If I fall short of perfection, I am a total failure. Making mistakes means I am worthless.

<u>Overgeneralization</u>—Generalising from a single negative experience and expecting it to hold true forever.
e.g. I got the presentation wrong. I'll never get it right. I botched up the interview. I'll never get the job I want.

<u>Negative Bias</u>—Focusing on the negative and filtering out all the positives. Only noticing the one thing that went wrong and ignoring all the things that went right.
e.g. It was a disaster...I played the wrong chord in the second verse of the song!

<u>Discounting the Positive</u>—Coming up with reasons why positive events don't count.
e.g. I got the part, but it was just luck.

<u>Jumping to conclusions</u>—Making negative interpretations without actual evidence as if you could read minds.

e.g. I could tell the audience hated it. Or, I just know something is going to go wrong.

<u>Catastrophising</u>—Expecting the worst-case scenario to happen.

e.g. Nobody is going to come to see the play. I am going to be so terrible at speaking, I will lose my job. They are going to think I am incompetent.

<u>Emotional Reasoning</u>—Believing the way you feel reflects reality.

e.g. I am really scared so I must be in danger. I feel worried I might fail, so I must be a failure.

<u>Demanding</u>—Holding yourself to a strict list of what you should and should not do and beating yourself up if you break your own rules.

e.g. I should be calm. I should play the piece without any mistakes. (If I don't, I don't deserve the job)

<u>Labelling</u>—Labelling yourself based on mistakes and perceived shortcomings. This is equivalent to putting yourself in a cage and throwing away the key.

e.g. I am a loser. I am an idiot. I am a failure. I am a mediocre speaker.

<u>Personalisation</u>—Assuming responsibility for things that are outside your control.

e.g. It's my fault the computer broke down in the middle of the presentation. I should have bought a better computer that doesn't break down.

In this hypnotic session, you will learn how to deal with catastrophic thinking effectively. It is now time to listen to your transformational hypnotic audio.

To do so, download the bonus package by typing the following link on your browser: https://tinyurl.com/daretobeseenonlinecourse

Alternatively, you can make up your own session. Begin by recording the induction and deepening as described in Chapter 6. Speak slowly and clearly into your recording device and then record the following points before finishing with the "awakening" section also described in Chapter 6.

Here is a summary of the online content:

Step 1: Induce hypnosis

Use an induction of your choice, remember your goal, and connect to your motivation.

Step 2: Connect to worst case scenario

Pick an event you have been catastrophising about. Think of the day when this event is scheduled for as a movie with a beginning, middle, and an end. In a moment, I want you to start watching this movie. Imagine that everything that could go wrong, goes wrong. For example, you have broken sleep, your kid has the flu, your boiler breaks down, you forget your phone at home, your partner is grumpy and it's simply not your day. Then you arrive at the event. Again, imagine that everything that could go wrong goes wrong, and turns out badly. Add any other negatives you can think of, perhaps you have shaking hands, a trembling voice, a stomach ache... Think of all the negative feelings you would experience; you might be sad, upset, in a crying mood. You may feel embarrassed or frustrated or even angry.

Step 3: Stop and reframe

Now, say to yourself, *"Even if all of this happened, I would survive. I would cope. The sun would still rise, it wouldn't be the end of the world. I would be ok."*
See yourself coping even with the worst-case scenario. Use humour, lighten things up, think of the funny side of even the worst circumstances (but don't make fun of yourself!).

Step 4: Relax

Now, the film has finished, so black out the screen, close an imaginary curtain, or see the scene fade into the background. Take three or more deep breaths. Take yourself to your peaceful place and relax until you feel calm.

Step 5: Choose empowerment

Now, choose a statement that empowers you. You can make up your own. These are a good starting point:
- *No matter what happens, I'll be ok.*
- *I choose to be in control of myself.*
- *I choose to create a better day.*
- *I choose to react positively to whatever happens.*
- *I know I can cope.*
- *I focus on what I want.*

Fill in the blanks: what is the outcome you want? A good beginning is to have fun!
Once you have chosen a statement that works for you, begin repeating it to yourself aloud until you really believe it.

Step 6: Create a new ideal scenario

Now, think of how you would ideally like the day and the event to go instead. Think about the way you would want to feel, act, and react to whatever may or may not happen. Imagine everything going perfectly.

By focussing on what you desire, you are giving your mind instructions to provide you with exactly that. You are choosing to attract the ideal outcome because what you move towards, moves towards you. So, fill in the details and make sure to connect to any and all positive feelings thoughts and ideas that accompany your success. You could even visualise these as a colour that you associate with the positive feeling you would like to elicit and imagine it spreading inside you. Bask in the glory of your success.

Step 7: Exit hypnosis

When you have spent enough time revelling in the good feeling you have created, count from 1 to 5, wiggle your fingers and toes, and open your eyes.

Repeat this session once a day for at least a week or until you begin to feel its effects. It will stop you catastrophising and empower you to feel calm, no matter what happens.

Homework Session 5

1) On an A4 sheet of paper, write down your rendition of the worst possible performance, presentation, interview, audition, or speech you could ever give. Allow yourself to be honest about your fears, and just go for it without editing. When you are done, go through the list of cognitive errors listed at the beginning of this chapter and underline all the cognitive errors you notice in your writing.
For example:

- *My presentation will go as badly as last time.* (Overgeneralization)
- *I will get my words wrong and it'll be a total disaster.* (Black and white thinking)
- *People will laugh and think I am a fraud.* (Catastrophising and jumping to conclusions)
- *I am so incompetent and stupid.* (Labelling)

When you have finished, use the objection technique to flip them around. (See the homework assignment in Bonus Session 2 for detailed instructions.)

2) Rewrite your day using positive language. Exaggerate and emotionalise. Remember your subconscious is like a smart eight-year-old. Use big, exciting words and use the present tense.
For example:
I wake up refreshed after a good night's sleep. I put a song on that makes me feel good. I visualise the performance going well and tell myself I am excited about it. I go to work and feel good about the opportunity I have been given to share my knowledge or song with my audience... (Keep going.)
You could use this to create a bespoke session for yourself by recording it as an autosuggestion. For more information on how to do this, read Chapter 6 and Bonus Session 3.

In the next chapter, we will look at how to let go of worry around performing situations so you can feel relaxed and give your best under scrutiny.

Audio Session 6

Letting Go of Worry

In this session, we will explore why we worry and how to let go of specific worries around performance.

Relax! Nothing is under your control

I don't know about you, but I want to make a t-shirt with this slogan. The problem with many of us is that we think we can only relax when everything is under our control, which is frankly, a suicide mission. I believe nothing *external* is under our absolute control and the more we try to assert control over what cannot be controlled, the more anxious we become.

Anxiety is exactly that: trying to control the uncontrollable and not controlling the controllable. In other words, the only thing we can truly have influence over is our reaction to events and situations. Control is only an illusion of safety, and it only gives temporary relief. It's never going to be enough, and the more you indulge in this coping mechanism, the more anxious and distressed you will become.

I'll give you an example. You may be worried about the audience's reaction to your 'performance'. You may be worried that some of them might not like you and may leave the room, or say something unkind. You may be worried you will be judged and rejected. You may try to avoid this by people pleasing or trying to guess what others may want from you, rather than being authentic. Or you may over-practice to reach perfection so that you cannot be found wanting. You may even worry that something technical could go wrong and leave you looking like a fool.

The problem with worrying about these scenarios is that there is no way you can control others' behaviours or circumstances. People are unpredictable and if you go down the route of avoiding anything that cannot be predicted, you will end up a recluse, safe in your inner inexpugnable tower and incredibly isolated.

The good news is that you can control your reaction to things by changing your perspective and judgement. You also need to learn to self-soothe. Anxiety is a habit fed by insecurity, which really translates as self-distrust. Oftentimes, we mistrust ourselves when we are confronted with stressful environments in which we feel vulnerable. If this happens to us, we will naturally try to find relief by learning coping mechanisms that will get us away from insecurity.

The two ways in which we typically react to these situations are:

- we attempt to control what might happen with worrying.
- we attempt to control what might happen with perfectionism.

Worrying is magical thinking

I remember hearing a story about a guy who would leave his house every morning right after breakfast and walk around his property three times. When asked why he did this, he would reply, "I am just making sure there are no tigers lurking around". Since he lived in Scotland, it seemed ludicrous that he would do this. When someone eventually told him his behaviour was crazy because there are no tigers in Scotland, he replied, "Of course there aren't. That's because of what I do!"

Most of us engage in worrying to prevent what might happen so we can feel safe. But does it ever work? Is it even possible? Or isn't it an act of magical thinking just like believing we are preventing tigers from appearing at our doorstep by circling the house three times a day? And if it's so crazy, why do we keep doing it?

Living unrehearsed can seem too scary an option. Instead, we anticipate what can go wrong in the false hope that we will be 'prepared'. I want to ask you a question: were you ever prepared for anything distressing that happened to you? Did worrying ever really help you, or did it just ruin your present and perhaps even set you up for a negative self-fulfilling prophecy?

Not only won't worrying help you if something wrong happens, but it will also make it more likely for that eventuality to manifest. This is not because of some magical force, but because when you only anticipate what could go wrong in life, you become convinced that you are doomed to failure. And when you think that way, your actions will attract failure.

Think about it. Imagine that you are shy or introverted and you become worried about going to an interview because you think the interviewers may think you are incompetent. If you indulge in fantasies where everyone on the panel looks strangely at you and judges you as inadequate, chances are when you reach the interview (if you even go), you will act in a way that will make them think you are indeed quite weird! You will get exactly what you were afraid of, simply because of your mindset.

In terms of the 'fight or flight' process, anxiety is a form of flight where you escape to a made-up universe where you feel safe and nothing 'wrong' could possibly happen. The problem is that kind of universe does not exist, and demanding control over life is like demanding to live in a place where only rainbows and unicorns exist.

The truth is that no matter how hard we try, we are confronted with uncertainty and unpredictability and the only way to navigate our way through it, is to accept that no matter what happens, we will be okay. The answer is not to try to avoid challenges, but to learn to trust that we can risk living life unrehearsed, spontaneously reacting to whatever may happen as it unfolds.

So, although you may trip just as you step on stage to give a big speech, it is how you react that matters. Will you choose to see it as proof that you are useless and incapable of doing a good job, or could you choose to laugh it off as a funny incident that makes you one with the rest of humanity?

Healthy thinking is a choice

The main point I want to make here, is that *healthy thinking is a choice*. It feels unnatural at first, because we are so used to thinking unhealthily that it has become automatic. Unhealthy thinking is thinking that focuses on shame and blame. It is the internalised critical bully who puts you down, dismisses you, shames you, blames you, and makes you feel small.

Healthy thinking focuses on kindness, compassion, and gentle encouragement. It is the internalised wise teacher who tells you the deeper truth, shows you solutions, and encourages you to keep going and to learn from your experiences in a non-judgemental way. Who you listen to and give energy to through the focus of your attention, is your choice. It takes practice to switch from *"shame and blame FM"* to *"gentle encouragement FM"*. It takes self-awareness to recognise you have been tuned into *"fear FM"* and decide to turn that off and switch to *"trust FM"*.

Which radio station would you rather listen to? You need to keep on switching channels every time you become aware that you've drifted back to the old frequency until eventually, the new habit becomes natural. Expect to feel frustrated at first. This frustration is temporary. Keep going.

How to deal with worry

Worrying is only helpful when it spurs you on to take action and solve a problem. If, on the other hand, you are preoccupied with what ifs and worst-case scenarios, worry itself is the problem. When you allow unrelenting doubts and fears to consume you, your emotional energy is sapped and your anxiety levels soar.

This can be paralysing and it can seriously interfere with your everyday life. But chronic worrying is a mental habit like any other, and you can break it by training yourself to stay calm and look at life from a more helpful perspective.

Nobody likes how worrying makes them feel, so why is it so hard to stop? The answer lies in the beliefs you have about it. Here are some common ones:

- Constant worrying will spiral out of control and drive me crazy or make me ill, but somehow, I can't stop myself.
- Worrying helps me avoid bad things. It helps me prepare for the worst and come up with solutions.
- Worrying shows that I care and that I am a conscientious person.

The trouble with the first belief is that worrying about worrying adds to the anxiety and keeps it going. This is similar to what happens when you worry about not being able to fall asleep. It keeps you awake.

The other two beliefs might seem positive, but the trouble is that they make it harder to give up worrying because you think that it is actually protecting you. Therefore, the first decision you need to make is to give up your belief that it serves a positive purpose. You need to realise that worrying is the problem, not the solution.

"But Elisa, telling myself to stop worrying doesn't work!" I hear you say. And I would reply, "Correct! This is because what you resist persists, remember?"

Trying to banish anxious thoughts makes them stronger, but this doesn't mean there's nothing you can do. You just need a different approach.

My method to successfully deal with worry has two different components:

1. Using a strategy of postponing worry combined with problem solving to empower you to change what you can change and let go of what you cannot.
2. Using hypnosis to construct metaphors that will help you let go of worry.

The first strategy will be outlined in the homework for this session. The second will be used in the transformational hypnotic audio that follows.

It is now time to listen to your transformational hypnotic audio recording.

To do so, download the bonus package by typing the following link on your browser: https://tinyurl.com/daretobeseenonlinecourse

Alternatively, you can make up your own session. Begin by recording the induction and deepening as described in Chapter 6. Speak slowly and clearly into your recording device and then record the following points before finishing with the "awakening" section also described in Chapter 6.

Here is a summary of the online content:

First, select a specific worry you have around performing.

Step 1: Induce hypnosis

Use an induction of your choice.

Step 2: Decision time

Decide it is time to see worry for what it is: an unhelpful behaviour. You are now going to let go of the specific worry you have selected.

Step 3: Letting go

Look at the metaphors listed below and choose one that particularly resonates with you. In the recording, I use Option 1, but if you feel you relate more to the other scenarios, feel free to go with a different option.

Option 1—Autumn leaves

Imagine you are in a beautiful autumn garden. Picture the time of day and engage all your senses in the feelings you experience as you walk on the grass. Imagine the brown and yellow leaves from the trees around you. The leaves represent all the worries you wish to dispose of.

Begin by raking all the leaves into one big heap. Take your time with this. When you are ready to let the worries go, imagine pouring gasoline on the leaves and setting them on fire. As you watch the smoke disappear high in the sky, feel yourself becoming lighter. When only the ashes are left, imagine you could collect them into a small bucket.

With the bucket in your hand, choose a spot where you will be planting a new seedling. Dig a small hole in the ground and imagine placing a seed at the bottom of it. Think about what this seed represents for you. This is the seed of a new you, what you could become, given enough nurturing and loving care.

When you have a sense of what that is, cover the ground again and sprinkle the ashes from the bucket onto it. Infuse the ground with your loving gaze, imagining the sun giving the seed all the energy it needs to grow in the coming days, weeks, and months.

Visualise what you'd like the seedling to grow into. Imagine it gently sprouting through the ground and eventually becoming a sturdy, beautiful tree. Proceed to step 4.

Option 2—The furnace

Imagine your body as a building with many rooms. Now, see yourself descending some steps to the basement. Here you will find a forge where you can see a glowing furnace burning hot with coals. Allow yourself to really fill in all the details of this furnace. Imagine what your eyes would see, what your ears would hear, and how it would feel to stand in front of such a hot fire.

When you are ready, imagine taking a blank piece of paper and a pen from your pocket. Note down the particular worry you want to dispose of. If there's more than one, you can use different pieces of paper for each worry.

When you have completed the task of writing, imagine scrunching up each piece of paper and ceremonially throwing them into the fire. Watch each piece burn and dissolve into nothing. Take pleasure in doing this. When nothing is left of the paper, close the door to the furnace and leave it behind you.

Next, see yourself walking upstairs to the very centre of the building where you will find a temple. Imagine this in any way that makes sense to you, making sure you engage all your senses in the process. This is a sacred place where your vision of the future is created and stored.

When you are ready, decide how you are going to impress your vision on the wall. Perhaps you could write down a sentence that encapsulates it like a sacred inscription. Or you could draw or paint a picture of your future on it. Alternatively, your vision might be a film that is being shown on a projector. Whatever method you choose, revel in the feeling you experience when you truly connect to the future you are imagining now. Proceed to step 4.

Option 3—Magnificent cliffs

See yourself walking on top of a magnificent cliff. You have been roaming through this landscape for quite a while when you realise you've been carrying a heavy load on your back. You are carrying a bag filled with stones which represent your worries.

Imagine that you want to proceed to the edge of the cliff where you can see the beautiful view of the sea stretching ahead for miles, but you can only walk slowly due to the weight you are dragging with you. See yourself arriving at the edge of the cliff with some effort, and stop there.

As you look at the breath-taking view, feel yourself making the decision that it is time to let go of your bag full of worries. You want to feel light and free to go onto the many adventures that await you. When you are ready, take the bag off your shoulders and deliberately let it drop into the sea.

Watch the bag as it plummets all the way down and disappears forever into the depths of the ocean. Feel the sense of freedom this gives you. When you can no longer see anything but water, you may want to bask in the light of the glorious sunshine all around you. Or maybe you could grow wings and fly away towards the horizon where the vision of your future awaits you. Proceed to step 4.

Option 4—Dirty laundry[16]

See yourself in a bathroom. Imagine filling up the bath with water. Imagine that your head has a trap door that leads to many loads of dirty laundry. The sheets and clothes inside your head are filthy and soiled. Those stains are the worries that you are now going to empty into the bath.

Dump your worries in the water and see it become dirtier and blacker as you do so. Stir the clothes until it is so black that you can no longer see the items inside the tub. What you are doing is letting go of what you no longer need.

Now, pull the plug and watch the black water flow down the drain. As the last drop disappears, notice how the items in the bath are now dry, bright, and clean. It's time to place them back into your head. Notice how good they feel and how fresh and clean they smell. Tell yourself that this feeling of lightness stays with you, even when you open your eyes. Proceed to step 4.

---

[16] This option is directly adapted from Cognitive Behaviour Hypnotherapist Adam Eason's work on anxiety.

Step 4: Time travel

Whatever option you have chosen, take a moment to imagine it's a year from now and you have achieved what you wanted by becoming the person you desired to be. With the abilities and experiences of the past integrated into the future, see yourself stronger than ever. Feel good about yourself and give yourself credit for all you have achieved. When you are ready, imagine you are looking back to the present. Reflect on how significant the decision you made to let go of worry has been in shaping the positive future you have created.

Step 5: Exit hypnosis

Drift back to the present feeling calm and refreshed. Now you have let go of worry, allow yourself to feel confident about your ability to create the future you desire. Expect it to happen and give yourself permission to feel excited about it. Count yourself out of hypnosis and do the exercise outlined below.

Homework Session 6

When you postpone worry, you are effectively breaking the habit of dwelling on worries so you can get on with what you want to do. You are not struggling to suppress your anxious thoughts. You are simply saving them for later.
So, rather than trying to cancel the worry, you are buying yourself a "moment of calm". In this moment, you have an opportunity to just be, because the part of you which wants to worry is satisfied, knowing

you'll do it later. As you develop your ability to postpone the anxious thoughts and resolve problems that are within your control, you will discover that you have more influence than you think.

Sometimes, worrying feels good because when you run through a problem in your head, you are distracting yourself from the unpleasant emotions you may have about the event. It may also feel like you are accomplishing something. But worrying is very different from problem solving.

When you problem solve, you evaluate a situation and come up with concrete steps for dealing with it. You then put into practice your plan and take action. When you worry however, you rarely find solutions. Keeping this in mind, proceed with the following exercise.

You will need:

- *A dedicated 'worry notebook'.*
- *A pen.*
- *Half an hour, every day, until you have mastered this technique.*

1. **Create a "worry period".** Choose a set time and place for worrying. It should be the same every day (e.g. in the living room from 5:00 to 5:20 p.m.) and early enough that it won't make you anxious right before bedtime. During your worry period, you're allowed to worry about whatever is on your mind. The rest of the day, however, is a worry-free zone.
2. **Postpone your worry.** If an anxious thought comes into your head during the day, make a brief note of it and then continue going about your day. Remind yourself that you'll have time to think about it later, so there's no need to worry about it right now.
3. **Go over your "worry list" during the worry period.** If the thoughts you wrote down are still bothering you, allow yourself to worry about them,

but only for the amount of time allocated for your worry period. If they don't seem important any more, cut your worry period short and enjoy the rest of the day.

What to do during your worry period

When the allotted time comes, open your worry book, and if you have any additional anxious thoughts about your performance, write them down. Identify the frightening thought. Be as detailed as possible about what you fear. Now, remember that these are not facts, but hypotheses that you are going to test. The idea is to challenge and examine these thoughts so you can develop a more balanced perspective. So, let's start by noticing if there are any cognitive errors present. You can find a list of cognitive errors in the previous session (Audio Session 5).
Now ask these questions:

- *Is the problem something you are currently facing or is it an imaginary "what if?*
- *If it is a 'what if?' what's the probability on a scale of 0 to 10 that it will happen?*
- *If the probability is low, what are some more likely outcomes?*
- *Is there a more positive and realistic way of looking at the situation?*
- *Is the thought you are looking at absolutely 100% true beyond any shadow of a doubt?*
- *Is the thought helpful?*
- *How will worrying about this help you? How will it hurt you?*
- *What would you say to a friend who had this worry?*
- *Can you do something about the problem or is it out of your control?*

Now, divide the page into two columns and fill each column

by dividing your thoughts and problems into things you can and cannot change.

Things I can change/ in my control	Things I cannot change/ out of my control
I am afraid I might not be prepared enough.	*People might now like the performance.*

What to do next:

Option 1—If the worry is about a problem you cannot solve

If the worry is about something you cannot solve, you need to tune into your emotions. Worrying helps you avoid unpleasant emotions by keeping you in your head. When you are in your head, you don't feel what's going on underneath. Although they will be temporarily suppressed while you worry, as soon as you stop, your negative feelings will return. Then you may start to worry about them: "What's wrong with me? I shouldn't feel this way!"

To stop this vicious cycle, you need to embrace how you feel. If this is scary to you, it may be because you believe you should always be rational and in control. Or because you think your feelings should always make sense. Or because you think certain emotions are not appropriate, such as fear or anger.

Try to accept that emotions, like life, don't always make sense. They are not always pleasant, but they are part of being a human. Let yourself experience them and trust that all that is needed is for them to be expressed.

Like water in a river, emotions need to flow. Trust that when you let yourself express even the most unpleasant of emotions, they will eventually become different and more manageable. Nothing lasts forever, and feelings shift and change like water. So, try to accept the items in the right-hand column and allow full expression of the feelings that emerge when you do.

As you observe them, imagine you are an outsider looking in. You are not reacting to or judging your feelings. Instead, you treat them like stormy clouds carrying heavy rain. You watch the storm come, and eventually pass. You are like a mountain, witnessing the weather without becoming stuck on a set of conditions. You don't engage; you observe instead, because it's only when you engage and hold on that you get stuck.

Option 2—If the worry is about a problem you can solve

If the worry is about something that can be solved—i.e. it's in the left-hand column—now is the time to start brainstorming. Make a list of all the possible solutions you can think of. Don't become too hung up on finding the perfect solution. Focus on what you have the power to change.

When you have finished brainstorming, pick the first item in the left-hand column, and ask yourself:

- *What first small step can I take in the right direction?*

Take action immediately. Once you have a plan and start doing something about the problem, you will feel a lot less worried. When you are done with this problem, move on to the next item on the list. When half an hour has passed, stop working; the rest can wait until tomorrow.

In the next session, we will reprogram your subconscious with the kind of mindset you need to enjoy being on stage. From staying in the present to enjoying the message you are delivering; this session will help you replace old patterns of negative self-talk with positive inner dialogue so you can truly thrive when performing in public.

Audio Session 7

Being Present

In this session, you will learn how to replace negative self-talk with positive, helpful inner dialogue so you can support yourself to give your best in any performance situation. You will also learn how to stay in the present and enjoy being heard and seen in your authenticity.

Performance anxiety takes you away from the present into an imaginary negative future. You worry about what might happen and what you will do about it. As a result, your performance will suffer greatly. This is because instead of focussing on what you are doing in the present, you are lost in your head, imagining futures that don't exist. When you do that, you are disconnected from what you are sharing and the audience will also become disconnected from you.

The solution to this is to stay focused on the now. A simple trick is to pay attention to your body sensations without judgement. This is because your body is *always in the present*. When you pay attention to the rhythm of your breathing—allowing for deep, slow breaths—you will be calming your body and slowing down.

Focusing on the present takes practice. At first, your mind will keep wandering off. This is normal. Accept the frustration as temporary. If a ship momentarily sails off course, all you need to do is correct the route. Every time you do this, you become more adept at noticing and correcting course. This process is part of the training. Negative self-talk is also the number one culprit when it comes down to anxiety and low self-esteem. Remember that your mind believes everything you tell it. So, when you say to yourself that you are a terrible performer or human being, your mind will believe it to be true. When you tell yourself that the audience is judging you and criticising you, your mind will believe it, too. You can counteract this by cultivating a habit of enjoyment and self-praise.

The best way to kick a bad habit is to replace it with a better one. The idea is to tell yourself you are already feeling the way you want to feel. When you engage in positive self-talk, you automatically remove all negative thoughts without trying. This feels unfamiliar at first, but as you keep repeating it and commit to make the unfamiliar familiar, it will change from something you do to who you are.

It is now time to listen to your transformational hypnotic audio. To do so, download the bonus package by typing the following link on your browser: https://tinyurl.com/daretobeseenonlinecourse

Alternatively, you can make up your own session. Begin by recording the induction and deepening as described in Chapter 6. Speak slowly and clearly into your recording device and then record the following points before finishing with the "awakening" section also described in Chapter 6.

Here is a summary of the online content:

Step 1: Induce hypnosis

Use an induction of your choice.

Step 2: Be open to possibilities

Open yourself to the possibility that you and your life could be very different. Open to change. Open to the possibility that past experiences might be holding you back, and that you could let go of this past conditioning and change to a new version of you; a version that's free to choose who you want to be.

Step 3: Replacing bad habits

When you are in hypnosis, your subconscious can learn and remember. However, your subconscious sometimes learns something and then applies it out of its context in time and place. Perhaps it learned a pattern a long time ago and although that was helpful back then, that behaviour is no longer relevant in the present. These patterns can be forgotten. We forget lots of things every day. Some we simply don't need; some we choose to forget. And you can start to choose to forget certain things that just don't work for you anymore.

Perhaps that old habit of worrying and negative self-talk might be one of those habits that you choose to forget. At first, you might need to remind yourself, just say to yourself: "I choose not to do this anymore". And as you do that, you will learn to start living in the present.

Maybe you've noticed worries and distracting thoughts when you were trying to concentrate during a performance in the past. And when we notice these worries and distracting thoughts, it is because our minds are not in the present, because both come from the past and the future, but never the present.

Step 4: Creating a positive future through the present

The past sometimes teaches us lessons that leave us hurt. And sometimes, we worry about old perceived dangers based on things that belong to the past. At other times, we worry about what might happen, looking into a crystal ball and worrying in advance. Tell yourself that as time goes on, you find yourself doing both less and less. This is because the past is gone. You can learn from the past but only at times that suit you. You are not the past, but you are turning your past into wisdom.

The future is yet to be created and you can create it positively and meaningfully by living in the present and allowing your actions and positive thinking to create your positive future.

And so, as time goes on, tell yourself that you will find yourself worrying far less; you will allow the past to remain in the past, your future to be created by your present, and as this happens, your will find your attention living in the moment. Since we create our present as we want it, from now on, you will choose the emotions that you want in that present moment, remaining calm, collected, and confident.

Step 5: Bring yourself back to the present

In the past, your subconscious mind has sometimes imagined the negative in situations. Maybe it has felt a little scared, and it's come up with ideas that represent its fears. For example, when you've been thinking of performing in front of others, sometimes your subconscious has come up with ideas about what might be scary. It's come up with ideas about what could go wrong, because it was a little bit anxious and it felt the need to fill in the gaps and imagine things that were a bit scary. But from now on, your subconscious can notice the truth in situations. And the truth—although always changeable—can very often be simple, supportive, and quite calm. From this moment onwards, when under the public eye—or whenever you are feeling fearful and overwhelmed, or you realise you're going over and over thoughts in your mind—your subconscious can start to realise that just as you can make yourself anxious, you can also calm yourself down. You calmly take some deep breaths and focus on your breathing and relax. You bring yourself back to the present moment and relax.

Tell yourself that no matter what may happen in the future, you can cope and you will survive. You could cope and you could bear it. Every time those old anxious thoughts try to return, remind yourself it is just an old habit. You come back to the present and you respond calmly and confidently, so you create the future you want, telling yourself repeatedly that you can deal with whatever may or may not happen.

You create your future by staying in the present and choosing the emotions you want in the present, remaining calm, collected, and confident. And every time you notice you are becoming tense or you are beginning to ruminate, remind yourself that you are becoming better at catching yourself and bringing your awareness back to the present. You bring yourself back to your peaceful place, you breathe deeply—and focus on your breath—and relax.

Step 6: Rehearse a new behaviour focused on enjoyment

Now, tell yourself that when performing, your subconscious can start to simply realise that the audience's aim is to enjoy themselves. That's what they really want. They are listening to you because they want to have a different experience and learn something new. That's what makes them want to invest their time in listening to you. They want to witness someone who is enjoying themselves so they themselves can enjoy the experience.

Tell yourself that the people who are watching you are just like you, and so they know what it is like to do something that is a little bit out of their comfort zone. It is the only way to really grow as a person and your willingness to do that is what they appreciate the most.

Remind yourself that the creativity and the enjoyment that you provide is a lot more important than any issues of perfection or technical knowledge. Your audience ultimately enjoys your presence and personality, and for them, someone who enjoys performing and who has passion, is worth investing their time in.

Your audience is there for positive reasons; they've invested their energy in coming along to appreciate your passion and your commitment—not to be perfect like some automaton that never makes a mistake, but as a person; a unique individual who is committed to share who they are, and who is passionate and expressive.

Imagine what it would be like to lose yourself in the experience of giving your speech, your presentation, or playing your instrument. See yourself enjoying your performance and remembering that the audience is on your side.

As you do this, you will be able to let go of any old negative experience of critical audiences—imagined or real—as you realise that if they ever had any niggles with your performance, it was out of their own insecurity or just because they were having a bad day and it had nothing to do with you. And you will remember that difference.

See yourself remaining calm and relaxed, able to enjoy the experience, and able to tap all that creativity, learning new skills so your natural personality is allowed to come to the fore.

And now think about each and every time you will be learning new skills when performing in the future. And make the decision now to remember that the audience are on your side, because there is only one side to have. From each day on, each time you listen to this recording, and each time you perform, tell yourself that it will become easier and more natural to simply enjoy being present.

From now on, each time you find yourself in a situation that stretches you out of your comfort zone, it will become more natural and easier for you to feel comfortable with it because your confidence in your abilities to learn will naturally increase, as will your abilities. By remaining calm, confident and relaxed you will be able to focus because you will no longer be distracted; instead you will simply be present and that will allow you to fully enjoy the experience.

As you learn new skills your natural personality and creativity will be allowed to come to the fore, and enable you to enjoy your experience. And you can find yourself being more relaxed and confident whenever you take on a new task because you know you are competent. You know what you are capable of doing, so as you take on tasks that you are capable of doing you can start to remember to take a deep breath and relax and just allow yourself the space in your mind to simply go ahead and do the task.

As you take on new challenges, you may surprise yourself to find that you can indeed do things you never imagined before. This makes you feel so proud of yourself, because every time you push yourself a little more, you discover new abilities and new talents you never thought you had, and you see that you are capable of much more than you ever imagined.

Allow yourself to become excited at all the new possibilities this opens for you, and all the new worlds of exciting opportunities for you to discover and enjoy. Imagine what these possibilities and opportunities that await you may include. Stay with the good feelings that you experience.

Every day we forget many things; any journey that we take we forget almost all of it before we reach our destination. And we're all on a longer journey, a journey through life in which we can forget all sorts of unhelpful facts and beliefs; all sorts of things can be discarded and before you realise it you can discard a lot those old patterns that are no longer helpful.

And so now on your journey you can start to decide what you remember and what you forget. And you can start to choose to remember the positives: those things that validate who you are, your qualities, your strengths. And you can start to dismiss and forget all those things in life that challenge our confidence, seeing them for what they are, unhelpful, not needed, best forgotten

And now, as you continue the process of relaxation, tell yourself that your subconscious mind is making all the changes that are necessary, in a way that only your subconscious mind knows how. It's like the tide ebbing and flowing, the changes just take place naturally. And some day in the future you'll look back and you'll be surprisingly delighted at just how easy it all was now that you've taken all this new learning on board.

Now remind yourself that every time you listen to your recording you will have a chance to rest, to relax, and simply to recover from any stresses and strains of life, your chance to just let go for a while. And while you benefit from that rest, your subconscious will learn and remember; your subconscious will take all it needs from the experience, sometimes taking something different, sometimes reinforcing the same, sometimes just learning better to forget.

Step 7: Exit hypnosis

When you are ready, count from 1 to 5 and exit hypnosis slowly. Now, proceed to the practical exercises outlined in the homework.

Homework Session 7

Here are some affirmations that you can use to train your positive self-talk. Choose the ones that most resonate with you or make up new ones. Feel free to modify them and personalise them. I strongly suggest you also make up your own affirmations specific to your situation. To know more about how to do that, read Bonus Session 3.

The following are general anti-anxiety affirmations. Repeat them aloud several times a day. One idea is to repeat them before going to bed or just as you wake up every single day for at least five times each.

Alternatively, you could use them as suggestions by recording an induction (see Chapter 6 for instructions) followed by your chosen statements. Experiment with second person versus first person, for example: 'the calmer I feel...' or 'the calmer you feel...' Some people respond better to one or the other. Include your name when possible.

You could also use your favourite affirmations as phone reminders so they pop up at regular intervals throughout the day.

Alternatively, write them down on a piece of paper you always carry with you or use them as a screensaver. Be creative. The important thing is to remind your subconscious that this is your new way of thinking. Keep going for a minimum of 7 days or more until they stick.

- The calmer I feel, the more I make wise choices.
- I am in charge of what thoughts I choose to pay attention to and this gives me control over how I feel.
- I am in control of how I react to situations that frighten me.
- I choose to imagine how I want to behave in any given situation.
- I expect the best and accept the rest.
- I focus on the present, one minute at a time.
- I create the future by focusing on the present as I want it to be.

- I choose the emotions that I want in the present moment: calm, collected, and confident.
- When I feel I am stressing myself out, I choose to calm myself instead.
- I remember I am in control of how I respond to situations that trigger me.
- When I feel afraid, I imagine how I want to behave in the situation I fear.
- I focus on the road instead of the wall. I focus on what I want.
- I remember that no matter what may or may not happen, I can deal with it and I will survive.
- No matter what happens, I'll be ok.
- When I feel tension, I take a moment to take a deep breath and relax.
- I relax into existence.
- I choose to find the serenity to accept the things I cannot change, the courage to change the things I can, and the wisdom to know the difference.
- I focus on the present.
- I choose to feel grateful for all the good things I already have in my life.
- When I feel anxious, I stop myself from flying into the future.
- I bring myself back to the present, noticing all the good things that are already in my life.
- I stop feeding my worries. I focus on creating what I want.
- I cross that bridge if and when I get there.
- I change what I can and I let go of the rest.
- No matter what happens, I can deal with it.
- I can and I will.
- I am master of my fate and captain of my soul.

In part IV of this book, we shall explore the successful performer mindset. You will learn to stop your automatic negative thoughts, stay in the zone under pressure, and increase your confidence. So, stick around and let's get going!

PART IV—
SESSIONS 8—10

THE SUCCESSFUL
PERFORMER'S MINDSET

DOWNLOAD the Dare to Be Seen BONUS PACKAGE

including a

FREE AUDIOBOOK, CHECKLIST and WORKBOOK

Templates, Training, Resources to Kickstart your Journey into Authentic Confidence under the Spotlight!

TO DOWNLOAD GO TO
https://hypnotichealing.co.uk/bonuses

Audio Session 8

Stopping your
Negative Thoughts

In this session, you will learn how to stop the automatic negative thoughts that come up in situations around performance you find stressful.

Sometimes, we are so used to responding to a certain set of circumstances with negative thoughts that they become habitual and natural. They become familiar. It is necessary to hone in on them and be aware of what these thoughts are so we can replace them with better ones.

Imagine there's two sides to your mind: one negative and one positive. One speaks to you with words such as, 'You are not good enough; you are going to fail'.

What does the other one say? Chances are the other one is a lot quieter and you are not accustomed to hearing it often.

As humans, we all suffer from a natural negative bias. It is a lot easier for us to be negative than positive, because negativity is wired into us so that we can avoid threats. So, we need to consciously counteract every negative thought with at least two positive ones to redress the balance.

We naturally dwell on the negative. Therefore, it is always important to have positive beliefs at your fingertips to remind yourself of the positive side of any situation daily. You always have a choice; you can indulge in negative thoughts and knock yourself out, or you can consciously focus on expanding your strengths.

Some people are afraid that self-praise will turn them into vain individuals who cannot see their own flaws. This could not be further from the truth. Arrogance is not the opposite of confidence. On the contrary, it is just another side of insecurity.

When you feel inadequate, you can either identify with that feeling and openly believe that you aren't enough, or if that is too painful, you can go into denial. When that happens, you will run away from the feeling of inadequacy by overcompensating.

You may run your life hunting for compliments or seeking approval from others as proof that you are adequate. You may chase achievements to prove you are worthy. You may become defensive whenever someone criticises you. This is not because you are confident, but because you are terrified of admitting that you could be found wanting. You are trying to prove to yourself that you are perfect and therefore beyond reproach, because you are secretly—and often unconsciously—worried that you are flawed and inherently worthless.

So, choose a situation in which you feel particularly anxious with regards to being in the public eye. Perhaps it's the moment you step on the stage or the podium. Perhaps it's the moment you sit down for your interview or audition. Perhaps it's the time you start your presentation.

Keeping this in mind, prepare to listen to your transformational hypnotic audio recording now.

To do so, download the bonus package by typing the following link on your browser: https://tinyurl.com/daretobeseenonlinecourse

Alternatively, you can make up your own session. Begin by recording the induction and deepening as described in Chapter 6. Speak slowly and clearly into your recording device and then record the following points before finishing with the "awakening" section also described in Chapter 6.

Here is a summary of the online content:

Step 1: Induce hypnosis

Choose an induction that resonates with you.

Step 2: Switch channels

Remember that you are the master of your thoughts. You don't have to allow negative thoughts to run away with you. You can learn to reduce them by giving more energy to the solution rather than the problem. Imagine that you are about to listen to the radio. You have a choice to tune into *"fear* FM" or into *"trust* FM". For too long, you have been tuning into the doom and gloom news. Where did that get you? It's time to switch the channel. So, imagine doing that.

From now on, tell yourself that you will only listen to the channel that gives you hope, encouragement, and praise. On this frequency, you hear beliefs that help you move forward; you constantly remind yourself of your strengths and you seek out opportunities to use them every day.

Tell yourself that you choose to engage in this new habit daily, hearing words of gentle reassurance that promote self-belief and self-trust. Now, let's put into practice the wisdom of the trust channel.

Step 3: Identify the negative

Imagine the situation where you typically experience negative thoughts. See it in detail as if you were there right now. As you do, talk to yourself in the way you normally would in this situation. Notice the kind of thoughts in which you typically engage. Tune into your feelings. Describe these feelings to yourself. Notice the kind of mental imagery you indulge in.

Step 4: Stop imagery

Now, imagine a huge bright STOP sign flashing right in front of you. Imagine a siren or alarm sounding—so intensely, it is impossible to ignore. Allow this imagery to engulf your attention fully and completely. Be creative and make the sign as vivid as possible and the sound as alarming as you can. The idea is that you catch the negative thoughts, feelings, and images associated with the triggering situation as early as possible. As soon as you do, interrupt them by using the stop imagery repeatedly. Practice this until you get the hang of stopping the negative thoughts in their tracks. This means you may have to run through this process a few times.

Step 5: Calm down

Engage in diaphragmatic breathing or any technique of progressive relaxation with which you are comfortable. You could take yourself to your peaceful place (see Audio Session 1 for instructions). You could imagine a colour you personally associate with calm enveloping your entire body. You could tell your muscles to soften and imagine what they would look like from the inside if they were loose and limp and relaxed. You get the idea.

Step 6: Create a new positive statement

Now that you are calm, think of a progressive positive statement that you are going to say to yourself instead of the old inner dialogue. Make sure this is something you want, not something you don't. Make sure the statement is positive and stated in the present tense. You could connect to your heart and ask your heart for help. If you are not familiar with this, refer to Audio Session 2 to learn how to do it.

Step 7: Rehearse the same situation with the new statement

Start repeating this power statement to yourself now while running through the scenario you chose at the beginning. Set this positive self-talk in your mind and make it convincing. Keep going through the scene a few times, reminding yourself of this deeper truth repeatedly until you feel you believe it.

Step 8: Review the process

Now, tell yourself that—every time you find yourself in the situation that previously triggered your negative thoughts as soon as you become aware of them—you will engage in the STOP imagery. You will then replace those old, unhelpful, toxic thoughts with positive, encouraging statements. Commit to practice this process for at least a week or for as long as needed to see results in how you feel.

Step 9: Exit hypnosis

Now, exit hypnosis and engage in the homework process.

Homework Session 8

Ask yourself these questions:
- *What would you say are your strengths when it comes to performing?*
- *What have other people said in the past you are good at?*
- *How often do you specifically think of these strengths daily?*

Write down the answers and make a list of your positive beliefs around performing. When you are done, ask yourself:
- *Which belief is going to help me move forward the most?*
- *Which is the most empowering?*

Select the most empowering belief and use it as your main affirmation.
Find opportunities to use your strengths during your next performance, interview, audition, speech, or presentation.

In the next session, we will explore how to deal with self-consciousness so you can easily get back into flow and perform at your best even when you get distracted.

Audio Session 9

From Self-Consciousness to Flow

In this session, you will learn how to get back into flow when you become momentarily self-conscious. Knowing how to deal with this common setback relieves the anxiety around it, helping you to feel more relaxed under pressure as well as making it a rarer occurrence.

The mind can only focus on one thing at a time. So, when you are focusing on the impact and the effect your performance will have on others, you cannot focus on the performance itself. When you are not paying attention to the activity in which you're engaging, you are not present but more than that, you are alienating both yourself and your audience.

Flow happens when you are entirely focused on what you are doing. When your attention is completely dedicated to the content you are delivering, you are allowing your subconscious to express that content automatically and effortlessly. It doesn't matter whether your performance is a song, a presentation, or a speech; when you're in flow, you are so absorbed in the subject matter that everything else ceases to exist.

When I am drumming, I must simply focus on the music I am playing and trust my arms and hands will do what they are supposed to without me consciously commanding them. If I start worrying about how well I am doing or how I am perceived, I will interfere with that process by interrupting it with my conscious mind. The only consideration that should be in your mind, is the activity you are performing.

You may not know this, but when children are complimented for engaging in an activity they enjoy, they become less confident doing it the very next time. This is because they are more likely to focus on the effect the action has on others, such as getting praise or rejection, rather than the internal feeling of enjoyment they had before. When you start thinking that others are assessing your work, the inner satisfaction of doing the work becomes tainted. You become distracted from doing itself and become self-conscious about how you are doing instead.

Self-consciousness happens when the focus of attention is directed on external considerations rather than the present moment and the activity itself. There is no space for winning or losing, passing, or failing, or looking good or bad during a performance. If these considerations suddenly intrude, you need to redirect your attention patiently and calmly to where it matters: the content you are passionate about sharing.

An ice-skating champion once described how she completely forgets where she is during important competitions. She is only aware of her immediate experience of skating. It could be a friendly rehearsal with a team member, or it could be a World Championship Final. It's only at the end of it that she reawakens to the reality of the tournament, the crowd, and the prize. She only gives herself permission to assess the quality of her own performance when it is over.

The idea is to become so single-minded that every time you give that speech, sing your song, or pitch your project, it's like it's the very first time you do it. You leave all distractions behind and you only think of the moment you are in. You focus on expressing the message you are sharing with all the passion you have for it. If distractions come, you calmly redirect your attention repeatedly to the message at hand, no matter how many times you must do it. Keeping all of this in mind prepare now to listen to your transformational hypnotic audio recording.

To do so, download the bonus package by typing the following link on your browser: https://tinyurl.com/daretobeseenonlinecourse

Alternatively, you can make up your own session. Begin by recording the induction and deepening as described in Chapter 6. Speak slowly and clearly into your recording device and then record the following points before finishing with the "awakening" section also described in Chapter 6.

Here is a summary of the online content:

Step 1: Induce hypnosis

Use an induction of your choice.

Step 2: Recall and rehearse flow

Recall what it is like to be in flow. Think of occasions when time disappeared and you were perfectly absorbed in the task at hand and all that mattered was the immediate activity in which you were engaged. See yourself becoming one with it. Whether it is a gig, audition, interview, presentation, or speech, imagine a time in the future when you are going to be performing, and imagine being in that same state of flow.

Step 3: Rehearse getting back into flow

If at any point you become self-conscious, that's ok. See yourself noticing it and remind yourself that what matters is the love you have for your subject. You want to share your message. You want the audience to fall in love with it the way you have. So, choose to focus back on the song you are singing, the feeling of the character you are playing, the love you have for the subject you are presenting, and the excitement you feel for the job offered. And when you do, everything else fades into the background automatically. The more you do this, the more you'll stay in flow, and the rarer will be the occasions when you feel self-conscious. Soon, it will become a faded memory of a habit you used to have.

Step 4: Behaviour replacement with the "Swish" protocol

Now, think of the old behaviour you want to replace. The old habit of thinking about external factors—for example, what other people think, or the result of your performance. You want to replace this with a habit of being absorbed in what you are doing.

So, picture, imagine, or sense that old behaviour you want to change. Make it a representation of what it is like to be distracted, worrying about the audience's perception of you, and watching yourself from the outside. See yourself behaving in this familiar way and put a picture frame around it. Then, move this picture to one side.

Now, create a new picture. See, imagine, or sense yourself behaving in the new way in the same situation. Make it a representation of what it is like to be fully focussed on the message you are delivering and sharing with your audience. Focus on the good feeling of enjoyment you experience when you do that.

Now, you have two pictures. Don't worry if you don't see actual images. You are not required to have hallucinations! It's enough to imagine them, feel them, or just sense them. The first picture is a representation of the old behaviour; the second is the new behaviour.

Now, take the second picture and shrink it down to the size of a stamp. Then bring the old picture—which may seem bright—back in the middle, and place your small, good stamp picture in the bottom right hand corner.

Now, darken the big bright old picture that represents the old behaviour and notice that the old picture is not as bright as it was; it's growing darker now, while at the same time, your new, better picture is growing bigger and brighter, until the old picture has disappeared completely.

Keep going and repeat this process five times until you can only see the good picture.

Step 5: Relapse control suggestions

Tell yourself that this is how you are going to behave from now on. If your old behaviour tries to return, take a deep breath, and say to yourself: "these feelings are only a reminder of how I used to feel". Notice how much time it has been since you felt the way you used to, and you will see that such times become increasingly rarer until they will eventually fade away and become only a faraway memory.

Step 6: Exit hypnosis

Count yourself out of hypnosis. Commit to repeat this session until you feel confident this is who you are now.

Homework Session 9

To reinforce the session, you can practice the "Swish" protocol using actual materials.

1. On a big piece of paper, draw a representation of your old behaviour. This could be symbolic or literal. Use colours that represent how you feel when you imagine behaving this way. Don't worry if you cannot draw or are not an artist. Even if you draw stick figures or just use symbolic imagery, it's what it means to you that is important. Alternatively, you could find an image in a magazine or online if you are more comfortable with that.

2. On another piece of paper, draw a representation of your new behaviour.

3. Take the first picture and blacken it with a dark pen or paint until you cannot see it anymore. All you can see now is a piece of paper that is completely black. When that is the case, burn it or bury it underground. Sounds extreme, doesn't it? Trust me, it will feel great!

4. Add bright colours and details to the second representation. Use colours that match how you want to feel when you behave like this. When you are done, put this picture on a wall where you can see it often.

In the next session, we shall look at how to increase your confidence during any performance so that nothing can ever stop you from sharing your talent with the world!

Audio Session 10

Increasing Confidence

Now it's time to really ramp up your confidence. In this last session, we are going to use anchors to help you release tension and feel really good about going on stage, giving that speech, or doing that interview. If you need a reminder of what an anchor is, please refer to Audio Session 1.

I will first show you how to effectively control your anxiety levels so you can learn to decrease them. After releasing physical tension, I will teach you how to connect and capture the confidence you felt during peak experiences in your life.

These experiences may be around performing or another area of your life. What matters is that there have already been occasions in which you felt competent and at ease. Now is the time to tap into those memories so you can use them to help you recapture that optimal state of mind and utilise it to enhance your future performances.

With this in mind, prepare now to listen to your transformational hypnotic audio.

To do so, download the bonus package by typing the following link on your browser: https://tinyurl.com/daretobeseenonlinecourse

Alternatively, you can make up your own session. Begin by recording the induction and deepening as described in Chapter 6. Speak slowly and clearly into your recording device and then record the following points before finishing with the "awakening" section

also described in Chapter 6.

Here is a summary of the online content:

Step 1: Induce hypnosis

Use a method of your choice to hypnotise yourself.

Step 2: Increase the tension

Imagine a performing situation where you might have felt anxious in the past, or you are worried you may feel anxious in the future. Really be there in your mind. Notice how you feel physically, and what your body is telling you. Rate your tension on a scale of 0 to 10 where 10 means as tense as possible, 0 means completely relaxed, and 5 is somewhere in between.

If the rating is less than 7, increase the tension by one point just by imagining it. Don't increase it by clenching muscles or holding your breath. Simply imagine it building. When you have spent enough time on this, go to the next step.

Step 3: Decrease the tension—fist anchor

Make a fist with your non-preferred, non-dominant, non-writing hand. Breathe normally and avoid tension in any other part of your body. Imagine all the tension in your body streaming down into your fist. Feel the tension flowing down to the fist, collecting in your hand, and leaving the rest of your body relaxed and comfortable.

When that has happened, take a deep breath in and as you exhale, release your fist quickly while throwing the tension away. It could be like throwing a ball into a pond or watching a balloon leave your hand and go up into the air.

Step 4: Create a circle of excellence

Now, take yourself to your peaceful place. See Audio Session 1 to learn how to do this. In your peaceful place, create a circle around you. See yourself sitting in the centre of your circle. This is your circle of excellence.

Tell yourself that the words 'my circle' are your post-hypnotic conditioned response—so, when you close your eyes and say those words in or out of hypnosis, you will be straight away back inside your circle.

Step 5: Peak experiences positive anchor

Now, allow a special memory to emerge. This is a memory in which you felt good about yourself. A time that gave you an inner sense of confidence. Perhaps you achieved something unexpectedly. Or you resolved a difficult problem. Or you overcame a challenge. It doesn't have to be a big deal. It could even be a memory of when you first learned to ride a bike!

When you have fully connected to this memory, relive the positive sensations as you experienced them then. Feel those confident feelings and inner strength flood back into you. Alternatively, imagine what it would be like if you had all the confidence you would ever need right now.

When you are connected to those feelings, make a fist with your dominant hand, and imagine them streaming down into the hand. When you can feel them in your fist, put this memory into your circle of excellence and relax your hand, knowing that from now on, whenever you make a fist with your dominant writing hand, these feelings will flood back into your consciousness, reminding you of what it's like to be confident.

Now, connect to a second memory that relates to a time you felt successful and competent—another situation in which you responded positively. Maybe you were complimented. Maybe you performed really well, or you did something that gave you a feeling of pride and self-belief.

Again, make a fist with your dominant hand and allow the feelings generated to flow into it. Then, place the memory into your circle of excellence and release the fist.

Repeat one more time with a third memory.

Step 6: Future rehearsal of connecting to your circle

Now, tell yourself that from now on, whenever you make a fist with your dominant hand, you will be reminded of these memories of success and you will connect to these feelings of confidence straight away. All you need to do is to imagine a circle in front of you. As you say the words 'my circle', step into it and make a fist with your writing hand; you will feel those good, strong, confident feelings fill you from the inside immediately.

Know that as you step into your circle increasingly often, you will also be able to add new experiences to it. There may be other memories springing to mind or new experiences resulting from your new-found confidence. You can add all of those to your circle to make it even stronger and more powerful.

Step 7: Combine anchors

Now, recall the previous situation where you felt anxious or worried and make a fist with your non-writing hand. Collect any tension in the fist and then release it.

Then, make a fist with your writing hand and imagine bringing all those good, positive, confident feelings and strengths into this new situation. Think about what it would be like to be able to deal with it in the way you wish, feeling strong and in control.

From now on, every time you notice feelings of anxiety or tension, tell yourself you will collect all the stress and fear in your non-writing hand by making a fist and then releasing it. And whenever you need your positive feelings of confidence, you will bring them to mind by clenching your writing hand.

Whenever you use your fists in this way, you will regain your feeling of being calm, focused, and in complete control and as you do, you will be confident and do well. The more you practice this method, the easier it will become.

Step 8: Exit hypnosis

When you are ready, count from 1 to 5 and come back to your full conscious awareness. Practice your anchors daily in and out of hypnosis. The more you do, the more powerful and effective the connection will be.

Homework Session 10

We learn by imitation. Others have trodden similar paths before, and as humans, we all have the same potential for growing and honing our skills. Modelling others is one of the fastest ways of accessing parts of ourselves that are present within us in embryonic form. Modelling is different from copying. You possess the same qualities you admire in others. If you didn't, you could not recognise them in anybody else.

Remember these people are not superhuman. They are just like you and me. At some point, they didn't have a clue what they were doing, but they committed to refining their craft and they became good at it. Talent is overrated; effort is a much bigger predictor of success. Let's get the process started right now.

1) Begin by identifying someone in your field that you admire for the qualities they possess. Perhaps they are excellent speakers, singers, musicians, actors, or presenters.

2) Make a list of the qualities they possess. Be as specific as possible and describe in detail how you know they have those qualities. You could ask yourself questions such as:

- *How do they move their body?*
- *How do they use their voice?*
- *What thoughts do you imagine they have?*
- *What do you imagine they would be saying to themselves as they step into the limelight?*

- *What do you imagine they would be saying to themselves when they make a mistake?*
- *How do you think they would handle failure?*

3) Now, the next time you are faced with a situation around performing in which you feel nervous, stop for a moment, and ask yourself:

- *How would (the person you admire) handle this?*

- *What would they do?*
- *What would they say to themselves?*

4) Pretend you are that person and experiment acting the way they would. You may be surprised to find you can access resources you never knew you had inside yourself. Like an actor stepping into his or her character's shoes, you may find those very qualities you admired in them being awakened in yourself.

In the next two bonus chapters, I will show you how to write your own affirmations and auto-suggestions so you can make self hypnosis fun and take it further.

Bonus 3

Letting Go of Limiting Beliefs

In this chapter, I will show you how to effectively use personalised affirmations and suggestions to let go of your limiting beliefs so you can take your performances to the next level.

You may have already heard of limiting beliefs, but what exactly are they? They are beliefs that limit your range of self-expression and experience. They are 'stoppers' that halt you in your tracks before you even start. They are disempowering and make you feel helpless. Here are some common ones:

- *I don't have enough money.*
- *I don't have time.*
- *I am not talented / pretty / young / slim / smart enough.*
- *I can't have what I want.*
- *I don't belong.*
- *People are mean / dangerous / against me.*

Although you may also share some of these, you will also have beliefs specific to you that stop you from being successful in the performing arena. It is important you address them directly. So, how do you know exactly which ones you have?

Find out what your limiting beliefs are

The fastest way to find out is to ask yourself the following questions:

- *What stands in the way of my (performing) success?*
- *What's stopping me from achieving what I want in this area?*

- *What do I think I am I not good at when it comes to performing in public?*

Write down the answers. These are your limiting beliefs around performing. Face your fears and be honest.

Now debunk them!

What you believe shapes your feelings and behaviours. Therefore, it is important to re-shape your beliefs to reflect the kind of experience you want to create in your life. When you have identified your limiting beliefs, it is time to transform them. Start by doubting their validity and debunking them rationally first. Take two of your worst disempowering beliefs and ask yourself:

- *How is this belief absurd or ridiculous?*
- *Who did I learn this from? Is this person worth modelling in this area?*
- *What will it cost me if I don't let go of this belief?*

Once you've created your beliefs, they will shape who you are. So, if you want to be better, you need to change your unhelpful toxic beliefs. The best way to let them go is to transform them into positive, empowering convictions. I will refer to these as affirmations or suggestions. The difference between the two is that affirmations are suggestions you say to yourself aloud or internally without the formal use of hypnosis. If, on the other hand, you decide to record the affirmations, you are effectively using self-hypnosis and I will call them suggestions.

To flip your limiting beliefs into affirmations, you can either follow the process described in Audio Session 2, or complete the "Hell vs. Opportunity" exercise described later in this chapter.

Do affirmations really work?

Some people complain that affirmations don't work. In fact, they say they make them feel worse. This is because if you don't follow some important rules when creating them, they may indeed produce the opposite effect.

There are two kinds of people when it comes to letting suggestions and affirmations in. Some people respond well to absolutely positive statements such as, "I am confident on stage" or "I love performing".

Others however, may well be put off by these kinds of statements and feel they just don't ring true. This will happen especially if you are new to affirmations and you are very used to talking to yourself negatively. If you are this kind of person, avoid writing absolutely positive statements.

Instead, use a 'progressive' style until you see positive results. Progressive affirmations suggest a state that is changing over time. So, for example "I am feeling more and more confident every time I am on stage" is a progressive affirmation.

These are the essential guidelines you should follow:

- Always use the present tense.
- Only use positive language (no "not" or "don't" or "won't").
- Be specific.
- Emotionalise (use words that suggest strong emotion).
- Exaggerate.
- Use progressive language when needed.
- Write suggestions you can believe.
- Imagine you are talking to a bright eight-year-old.
- Focus on what you desire, not what you don't want.

The hell versus opportunity exercise

Now, let's start transforming those go-to negative limiting beliefs you identified above.

Take a piece of paper and divide it into two columns. Name the first column 'Hell' (or if you prefer you can just say 'limiting beliefs') and write down the words you usually say to yourself when speaking about this particular challenge: "*I am the worst speaker, I am incompetent, I am not good enough, I always botch up interviews*".

Now, name the second column 'Opportunity' and for every negative belief, come up with an alternative set of words that you can use to replace the first set. This is what your response is going to be when the negative thoughts emerge. Make sure you word your sentences in a way that makes you truly believe them. If necessary, use progressive words.

Remember, this is about choosing a better, more useful perspective, taking responsibility for change, and clearly telling your mind what you want (not what you don't want) with positive words, in the present. It's about telling your mind you can change regardless of your past.

When you phrase your suggestions or affirmations, you can address yourself either in the first person, for example, "I am…." Or in the second person, such as "You are…"

There are studies that suggest that using the second person can be more powerful, especially when used in conjunction with your given name. So, if your name is Kathy, you may write something like: "Kathy, you are a wonderful speaker!". However, I suggest you experiment and see what works best for you.

For example:

HELL (LIMITING BELIEFS)	OPPORTUNITY (EMPOWERING BELIEFS)
I always forget the lyrics of my songs.	*My memory is perfect; words flow automatically and easily.*
I worry about making mistakes.	*Creativity is more important than perfection.*
I am distracted by people in the audience.	*I focus on the song; I fall in love with the song, and make the audience fall in love with it, too.*
What if the audience thinks I am incompetent?	*The audience is on my side. They want me to do well. They enjoy themselves when I enjoy myself.*
I hate performing.	*The more I perform, the better I become, and the more I love it.*

Once you have this set of alternative statements, start challenging yourself. Use them in your daily life by either saying them aloud or internally, as thoughts. Either use these as self-hypnosis suggestions, or read your 'opportunity' affirmations aloud every day for a minimum of 7 days or until you feel they have become a core belief.

How to use affirmations properly

When:

If you decide to use affirmations, I would recommend you choose one belief that feels most relevant or a set of related beliefs at any one time. Repeat it to yourself, preferably before bed. This will help you go to sleep with a good frame of mind and allow for relaxation which, in turn, aids good sleep.

Another reason for repeating affirmations at night is that early morning REM phase dreaming helps grow new connections in the brain. Information acquired just before sleep is integrated especially well. If you repeat your affirmations in bed, you are helping to wire them deep into your system.

How:

The way to repeat the affirmations is also important. Don't just say them. Mean them. Imagine them. And most importantly, feel them. Remember, your subconscious responds to strong emotion. What would it be like to believe them to be true? What would it feel like if they were already a reality? Connect to the emotions you would feel. Choose to trust what you want is on its way.

How often:

The amount of repetition is also important. New habits are formed through repetition. I would suggest you repeat each affirmation to yourself *slowly* either aloud ten times, or silently twenty times. Saying something aloud makes it real and it is less likely you will be distracted by other thoughts, so if you choose to say the affirmations to yourself silently, you will need to repeat them more often.

The number of times I suggest here is not mandatory, but it is based both on the power of ritual and on ease of recall. Practicing silently before sleep may make you fall asleep, so if you choose to repeat them inwardly, I would suggest you count the times you are saying your affirmation using the fingers of both your hands. As you go through your hands twice you will have twenty affirmations done!

Repeating these phrases may feel unfamiliar, but stick with it. Initially, it will be a choice, something you decide to do. But eventually, it will start to become part of who you are. The more you practice this, the easier it will become, and the easier it becomes, the more you will want to do it. You are wiring your mind to move towards success instead of coming up with obstacles and resistances.

Other ways of using them:

Another way of using affirmations is to scatter them everywhere for you to see during the day. Here are some possibilities:

- You could create a reminder on your phone or turn them into a screensaver.
- You could pin them under your fridge magnet.
- You could write them on a card and put them in your wallet.

Remember to stop every time you see them and really connect to what they mean. Imagine how you'd feel if your affirmation was already a reality, and treat it as such.

If you write your affirmations on a card, always remember to bring it with you so that when you suddenly feel anxious or have a nagging negative thought, you can take the card out and say the affirmation aloud. This will snap you out of your current negative loop and help you switch on to a more helpful one that brings you closer to your goals and makes you feel good.

Using suggestions with self-hypnosis

When you are making a self-hypnosis mp3 recording using suggestions, either record a 5 to 10-minute silence before you start repeating your suggestions, or record your induction first. Refer to Chapter 6 and use the induction provided following the rules outlined.

As for affirmations, always focus on one type of suggestion at a time. When you use self-hypnosis, it is good to drive the point home by repeating different versions of the same suggestion, thereby expressing the same concept from slightly different angles, but always ensuring the theme is the same.

You will get the best results by focusing on one issue at a time and not jumping to the next point of focus until the current one has been absorbed.

Creating affirmations and suggestions doesn't have to be boring. Make it fun! If you want to be creative and do something a little different, I invite you to read the next chapter on how to use poems for mind mastery.

Bonus 4

Poems for Mind Mastery

In addition to traditional affirmations and suggestions, it can be fun to write short, evocative poems to help train your mind to focus on what you want when you start engaging in self-hypnosis. Remember, the mind responds to imagery and metaphor more than analytical language. That is why a poem, like a still photograph, can speak a thousand words.

Your poems don't have to be perfect. This isn't about creating a piece of literature. It is to help you connect to the deeper truth of your purpose, your performance, and how you want to share your message with others. I made up some poems here to give you an example. I invite and encourage you to make up your own.

Perfect performance
Time stops
Deeply rooted
I stand witness
To the rhythm
Of my song
A hollow reed
An empty channel
I stand witness
To the stillness
Of my voice
Now I surrender
I am just a mirror
I stand witness
To the struggles
Of the world

DARE TO BE SEEN

I am the messenger
The Gods' interpreter
I stand witness
To their riddles
And their jokes

Stopping thoughts
Crystal clear
Shines like a rainbow
Clouds dispelled
Blown away by wind
Stopped like a clock
When the finger points
In a still iced drop
I say stop!
And the screen goes lucid
I say stop!
And the screen freezes up
Thoughts as leaves, blown away by water
Thoughts as leaves, washed away by rain

Command of thoughts
Laser beam focused on a dot
Future point the direction's hot
Thoughts like arrows on appointed spots
Thoughts like bullets make the questions drop
Thoughts as faithful soldiers of the mind
Thoughts as dutiful slaves of mankind
Thoughts my servants I wave my magic wand
I am the boss in control, flow at my command!

Witness to thoughts
Thoughts
Like waves they break on shore
One small, outstretched, shying away, closed
The other open, wider, shows its might and goes
Like a fisherman on a dock
Absorbed in the movement of water
I reach down inside the silence
Pick up one fish and let it go
Pick up another and rejoice for a moment
Pick up a last one and bring it back home.

It's now time to make up your own poem and use it either as an auto suggestion or an affirmation. Remember to have fun and enjoy the process as much as you can!

Conclusion

Congratulations! You have made it! You have committed to the process of learning how to use your brilliant mind to overcome performance anxiety for good. You are now well on your way to finding new joy doing what you love and sharing it with the public.

However, remember to keep up with the mental fitness regime you have undertaken! Like any other fitness regime, this is a lifestyle change that you need to cultivate every day. So, if at any stage you need a refresher, go back to the particular session you need to revise and go through it again.

It is important to keep the mental muscles active, just like you would any physical ones. If you don't use it you lose it, so keep using them! As a matter of principle, I urge you to commit to your mental and emotional wellbeing. Make it a priority. Get out of your comfort zone every day and keep expanding it. Do something that makes you a tad nervous every day and your tolerance for new, exciting situations will become higher.

Commit to learning from those who have gone before you, and from your peers. I would strongly suggest you record videos of your performances or rehearsals if you can and if it is applicable to your situation. Then, watch yourself with a constructive eye. This means that you notice the things you did right first and then gently suggest improvements.

Next time, focus on those improvements and rehearse again. You can also ask others for constructive feedback, but make sure they are the kind of people that you can trust, so you don't end up with a bunch of negative advice.

If you haven't already, consider joining my Facebook support group, *Master the Stage*, which is connected to my online course, *Dare to be Seen* . You can find the course by typing the following links into your browser:

https://tinyurl.com/daretobeseenmasterclass
Most of all, shine your light on the world! Trust me, it needs it.

About the Author

Elisa Di Napoli has been in full time clinical practice as an integrative hypnotherapist and coach since 2001. Practicing in both New Zealand and Scotland, her work places a great deal of importance on positive mental health, Neuro Linguistic Psychology, and Holistic Coaching. She originally studied philosophy 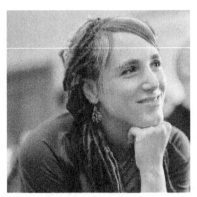 and comparative religion, but took up hypnotherapy after an interest in shamanism led her to explore the mind-body connection within altered states of consciousness.

She studied hypnotherapy in America at the prestigious Hypnotherapy Training Institute of Northern California known as one of the first licensed hypnotherapy schools in the world where she learned from the teachers of the teachers Randal Churchill and Ormond McGill. She also studied cognitive behaviour hypnotherapy and hypnotic coaching at the Anglo European College of Therapeutic Hypnosis.

Coming from a diverse background including philosophy, art, comparative religion, music performance and acting she has a Graduate Diploma in Electronic Music Composition and Performance as well as a BA (Hons) in Comparative Religion at the University of London. She is a drummer and an accomplished singer-songwriter with twenty years performance experience and eleven albums under her belt.

She is passionate about learning and has been involved in many drumming groups, improv comedy classes, performance workshops, drama, and clowning classes. When she is not making music, writing, or taking courses, she greatly enjoys the company of her dear cat, Bubulina

Therapy and coaching: www.elisadinapoli.com
Music: www.elyssavulpes.com

If you liked this book please leave a review by going to
https://elisadinapoli.com/dare-to-be-seen-book-review/
and tell me what you think.

Thank you!

**REGISTER for the Dare to Be Seen
FREE MASTERCLASS**

Discover

3 SECRETS TO STOP STAGE FRIGHT AND PERFORM WITH AUTHENTIC CONFIDENCE EVEN IF YOU ARE NOT AN EXTROVERT

Templates, Training, Resources to Kickstart your Journey
into Authentic Confidence under the Spotlight!

TO DOWNLOAD GO TO
https://tinyurl.com/daretobeseenmasterclass

Made in the USA
Coppell, TX
19 December 2021